Preface

One of the vital functions of emergency medicine is to differentiate between those who need emergent treatment from those who don't. Primary methods of differentiation across test-treatment thresholds include a detailed history and physical examination, and clinical judgment. The skills of taking a history, doing a physical examination, and clinical judgment are developed through medical school, residency, and the experience of evaluating and treating patients. Another primary method to differentiate patients who need emergent treatment is the use of diagnostic testing. The technology of testing in emergency medicine has blossomed in the past 50 years and continues to change rapidly with a greater availability of advanced radiography (CT, ultrasound, and MRI) and novel laboratory tests. There has also been a proliferation of research studies designed to guide test ordering and application of test results to individual patients. However, not all patients in the emergency department necessarily need tests. Many disease processes can be excluded reliably by clinical criteria alone. Probably the best example of this is ankle sprains, where only a small proportion of patients will have radiographs that demonstrate clinically significant fractures. Clinical decision rules for diagnostic testing can serve as guides in deciding which patients may not benefit from testing in the emergency department. Because the art and science of diagnostic testing is so central to emergency medicine practice, emergency physicians must be experts in this area.

The purpose of this book is to present relevant questions on diagnostic testing that arise in everyday emergency medicine practice and to comment on the best available evidence. The first part of the book serves as an overview of the science of diagnostic testing and reviews the process behind the development of clinical decision rules. Subsequent chapters focus on practical questions that have been addressed in original research studies. We provide a review of the current literature on a specific question, an interpretation of the clinical question in the context of the literature, and finally how we apply the evidence to the care of our patients. Importantly, we also provide the actual data, sample sizes, and statistics. As readers, you can come to your own conclusions about how to interpret the best available data by understanding not just the bottom line study conclusions but also the limitations of study designs. As a caveat, our comment section should not be interpreted as the standard of care. Not all emergency departments have the same resources for testing or treatment, nor do all departments have the same availability of specialty consultation. Therefore, it is vital to evaluate our interpretation of the literature in the context of your local resources and practice patterns.

Jesse M. Pines
Worth W. Everett
2008

Foreword

Open any copy of the *Wall Street Journal* and read "What's News" on the front page. You will consistently learn about the status of new drugs, vaccines, medical devices and equipment that will impact human medicine. The headlines often recapitulate some version of this story: "Trial Hints of Promise for New Cancer Drug." Diagnosis does not make headlines. It could be reasonably asserted that both lay and medical society alike afford excessive attention on treatment of disease, rather than its detection. After all, since when did the rich family travel across two states to bring dad to the Mecca ". . . to get the best evidence-based decision rule?" Alas, decision rules and clinical diagnosis are the linemen on our metaphorical medical team. They block and tackle, but they seldom dance in the end-zone or make the highlights.

However, the next 40 chapters illuminate the importance of clinical criteria to screen for emergency conditions. Taken as a whole, this text shows that decision rules do not just sort out presence or absence of disease, but help direct the use of resources, and ultimately vector patients toward the correct place in the mind of the clinician. What does that mean? From a treatment standpoint, all that matters is what the clinician formulates a correct belief. If he or she believes a patient has a disease, then treatment and its benefit will follow. Conversely, if the clinician rejects the belief that a disease is present, the patient will be spared the risk of unnecessary treatment. Taken in its parts, each chapter presents a comprehensive, contemporaneous presentation of the published decision rules that matter in emergency medicine. The authors invoke a friendly and no-nonsense style of writing, and they employ clinical examples that make these criteria spring to life. The authors paint the picture of how these criteria fit into the overall complex process of human decision-making at the bedside, and I believe this text will help emergency clinicians take the safest, fastest, cheapest route to arrive at the correct belief about need for treatment.

Like all humans, most ED physicians have personalities that embody different characteristics at different times, ranging from the erudite academician to the wise-cracking "pit doc." This book will serve this range of need very well. As a researcher in this field, I believe this work will serve a vital role to help me understand-and perhaps explain-the theoretical construct of clinical decision rules in modern emergency medicine. As a pit doc in the ED, I expect this book will become my dog-eared companion that I will open and read aloud on most shifts. Allow me to suggest that the subject of each chapter appears in cadence, one after the next, in a way that resembles the chief complaints that pop up on your ED patient tracking system during any given shift. If for no other reason, this work will retain importance because of the brut workload and time required to organize, discuss and reference these decision rules and related criteria under one cover.

I am still waiting for the headline: "New Decision Rule Saves Lives and Money," and I will probably be waiting for a while longer. In *Evidence-Based Emergency Care: Diagnostic Testing and Clinical Decision Rules,* Pines and Everett have turned up the voltage to the spotlight, and aimed at the process of screening and diagnosis in the emergency department. Keep a copy nearby for your next shift.

Jeffrey Kline
2008

Evidence-Based Emergency Care

Diagnostic Testing and Clinical Decision Rules

Jesse M. Pines, MD, MBA, MSCE

Assistant Professor, Department of Emergency Medicine
Senior Scholar, Center for Clinical Epidemiology and Biostatistics
University of Pennsylvania School of Medicine
Philadelphia, USA

Worth W. Everett, MD

Assistant Professor, Department of Emergency Medicine
University of Pennsylvania School of Medicine
Philadelphia, USA

Blackwell
Publishing

BMJ|Books

This edition first published 2008, © by Jesse M. Pines and Worth W. Everett

BMJ Books is an imprint of BMJ Publishing Group Limited, used under licence by Blackwell Publishing which was acquired by John Wiley & Sons in February 2007. Blackwell's publishing programme has been merged with Wiley's global Scientific, Technical and Medical business to form Wiley-Blackwell.

Registered office: John Wiley & Sons Ltd, The Atrium, Southern Gate, Chichester, West Sussex, PO19 8SQ, UK

Editorial offices: 9600 Garsington Road, Oxford, OX4 2DQ, UK
     The Atrium, Southern Gate, Chichester, West Sussex, PO19 8SQ, UK
     111 River Street, Hoboken, NJ 07030-5774, USA

For details of our global editorial offices, for customer services and for information about how to apply for permission to reuse the copyright material in this book please see our website at www.wiley.com/wiley-blackwell

Library of Congress Cataloguing-in-Publication Data

Pines, Jesse M.
  Evidence-based emergency care : diagnostic testing and clinical decision rules / Jesse M. Pines, Worth W. Everett.
    p. ; cm.
  Includes bibliographical references.
  ISBN 978-1-4051-5400-0
  1. Emergency medicine—Diagnosis. 2. Emergency medicine—Decision making. 3. Evidence-based medicine. I. Everett, Worth W. II. Title.
  [DNLM: 1. Emergency Medicine—methods. 2. Diagnostic Techniques and Procedures. WB 105 P649 2008]
  RC86.7.P56 2008
  616.02'5—dc22   2007043480

ISBN: 978-1-4051-5400-0

A catalogue record for this book is available from the British Library.

Set in 9.5/12pt Minion by Graphicraft Limited, Hong Kong
Printed in Singapore by Utopia Press Pte Ltd.

1   2008

Contents

About the Authors

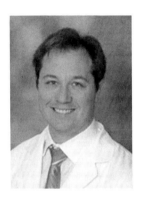

Jesse M. Pines, MD, MBA, MSCE is an Assistant Professor of Emergency Medicine and Epidemiology at the University of Pennsylvania School of Medicine and a board-certified emergency physician. He is a Senior Scholar in the Center for Clinical Epidemiology and Biostatistics and Associate Director of the Emergency Care Policy Group in the Department of Emergency Medicine. He holds a Bachelor of Arts and a Masters of Science in Clinical Epidemiology from the University of Pennsylvania as well as a Medical Degree and Masters of Business Administration from Georgetown University. He completed a residency in emergency medicine at the University of Virginia and a fellowship in research at the Center for Clinical Epidemiology and Biostatistics at the University of Pennsylvania. He lives in Wynnewood, Pennsylvania with his wife Lori and two dogs.

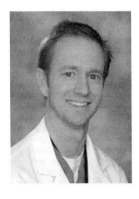

Worth W. Everett, MD is an Assistant Professor of Emergency Medicine at the University of Pennsylvania School of Medicine and a board-certified emergency physician. He holds a Bachelor of Science degree from McGill University and received his Medical Degree from the University of Texas-Houston. He completed a residency in emergency medicine at the University of California-Irvine in 2000. He now lives in Bellingham, Washington with his wife Linda and two children, Vail and Amelie.

SECTION 1
The Science of Diagnostic Testing and Clinical Decision Rules

Chapter 1 **Diagnostic Testing in Emergency Care**

As providers of emergency care, we spend a good deal of our time ordering and waiting for the results of diagnostic tests. When it comes to determining who needs a test to rule out potentially life-threatening conditions and subsequently interpreting test results, we are the experts. We are experts at diagnostic testing for many reasons. First and foremost, we see a lot of patients. The expectation, especially if you are working in a busy hospital, is that you see everyone in a timely way, provide quality care, and make sure patients are satisfied. If we order time-consuming tests on everyone then emergency department (ED) crowding will worsen, efficiency will decline, the costs of care will go up, and patients will experience even longer waiting times than they already do. However, differentiating which patients truly need tests in the ED is a complex process. Over the past 30 years, scientific research into diagnostic testing and clinical decision rules in emergency care has advanced considerably. Now, there is a greater understanding of the sensitivity, specificity, and overall accuracy of tests. Validated clinical decision rules provide criteria whereby many patients do not need tests at all and serious, potentially life-threatening conditions such as intracranial bleeding and C-spine fractures can be ruled out based on clinical grounds. There are also good risk stratification tools to determine the probability of disease for conditions like pulmonary embolism before any tests are even ordered.

So how do we decide who to test and who not to test? There are some people who obviously need tests, such as the head-injured patient who has altered mental status and who may have a head bleed. There are also those patients who obviously do not need tests, such as patients with a simple toothache. There is a large group of patients in the middle where testing

Evidence-Based Emergency Care: Diagnostic Testing and Clinical Decision Rules. By J.M. Pines and W.W. Everett. Published 2008 by Blackwell Publishing, ISBN: 978-14051-5400-0.

decisions can sometimes be challenging. This group of patients is where you may find yourself to be 'on the fence' with regards to testing. It may not be clear whether to order a test, or even how to interpret a test once you have the results. And finally, when we receive the results of a test that is not what we suspected clinically, it may be unclear how to extrapolate from the test results to the care of that particular individual patient.

Let's give some examples of how diagnostic testing can be a challenge in the ED. You are coming onto your shift and are signed out a patient for whom your colleague has ordered a D-dimer test (a test for pulmonary embolism). She is 83 years old and developed acute shortness of breath, chest pain, and hypoxia (room air oxygen saturation = 89%). She has history of prior pulmonary embolism and physical examination is unremarkable except for mild left anterior chest wall tenderness and notably clear lung sounds. The test comes back negative. Has pulmonary embolism been satisfactorily ruled out? Should you perform a pulmonary angiogram or a computed tomography (CT) scan of the chest, or maybe even consider a ventilation/perfusion (V/Q) scan? Was D-dimer the right test for her to begin with?

Let's consider a different scenario. How about if a D-dimer was ordered on a 22-year-old male with atypical chest pain and no risk factors, and the test comes back positive; what do you do then? Should he be anticoagulated and admitted? Does he have a pulmonary embolism, or should you move forward with further confirmatory testing before initiating treatment? Or is he so low risk, that he's probably fine anyway? But you could argue, if he was so low risk, why then was the test ordered in the first place?

In another example, you are evaluating a 77-year-old female who has fallen down and has acute hip pain and is unable to ambulate. The hip radiograph is negative. Should you pursue it and possibly get a CT or magnetic resonance imaging (MRI) scan done? But the test is negative so can't she go home?

These are examples of when test results often do not confirm your clinical suspicion. What do you do in those cases? Should you believe the test result or your clinical judgment before ordering the test? Were these the optimal tests for these patients in the first place? Remember back to conversations with your teachers in emergency medicine on diagnostic testing. Didn't they always ask: "how will a test result change your management?" and "what will you do if it's positive, or negative?"

The purpose of diagnostic testing is to reach a state where we are adequately convinced of the presence or absence of a condition. Test results are interpreted in the context of the prevalence of the suspected disease state and the clinical suspicion of the presence or absence of disease in the individual patient. For example, coronary artery disease is common. However, if we look for coronary disease in 25 year olds, we are not likely to find it because it is very uncommon in that population. There are times when your clinical suspicion is so high that you do not need objective testing. In those patients, you can proceed with treatment. Other times you do need testing to confirm what you think is the diagnosis or to rule out more severe, life-threatening diseases.

The choice over whether to test or not test in the ED also depends upon the resources of the hospital and on the patient. Some hospitals allow easy access to radiographic testing and laboratory testing. In other hospitals, obtaining a diagnostic test may not be so easy. Some places do not allow certain types of tests at night (like MRIs and ultrasounds) because staff may be unavailable to perform them. Sometimes a patient may not necessarily need a test if you believe they can be trusted to return if symptoms worsen. For others, you may believe that a patient's emergency presentation may be the only time that they will have access to diagnostic testing. For example, saying to a patient "follow-up with your doctor this week for a stress test" may be impractical if the patient does not have a primary care doctor or does not have good access to medical care. You may practice in an environment where you cannot order a lot of tests (like developing countries). You also may be in an office environment that simply does not have easy access to testing. However, regardless of the reason why we order tests in the ED, what is certain is that the use of diagnostic testing in many cases can change how you manage a patient's care.

Sometimes, you may question your choice of whether to test, to not test, or whether to involve a specialist early. Should you get a CT scan first or just call a surgeon in for a young male with right lower quadrant pain, fever, nausea, and possible appendicitis? How many cases have you seen where the CT scan has changed your management? What if it is a young, non-pregnant female? Does that change your plan?

How about using clinical decision rules in practice? By determining if patients meet specific clinical criteria we can choose not to test if they are low risk. Do all patients with ankle sprains need X-rays? Can you use the Ottawa Ankle Rules in children? What are the limits of clinical decision rules? Is it possible to apply the Canadian C-spine rules to a 70-year-old female? These questions come up everyday in emergency medicine practice.

In fact, a major source of variability among physicians is whether or not they order tests. Remember back to your training when you were getting ready to present a patient to the attending physician. Weren't you trying to think to yourself: what would she do in this case? What tests would she order?

Access to test results helps us to decide whether to treat the disease, initiate even more testing, or no longer worry about a condition. As emergency physicians, we gain confidence in this process with experience. Much of the empirical science and mathematics behind the testing described in this book becomes instinctive and intuitive the longer you practice emergency medicine. Sometimes we may think a patient does not need to be tested because the last 100 patients who had similar presentations all had negative results. Maybe you or a colleague were 'burned' once when a subtle clinical presentation of a life-threatening condition was missed (like a subarachnoid hemorrhage). The next patient who presents with those symptoms is probably more likely to get a head CT followed by a lumbar puncture. Is this evidence-based?

Step back for a moment and think about what we do when we order a test. After evaluating a patient, we come away with a differential diagnosis of both the most common and also most life-threatening possibilities. The following approach to medical decision making was derived by Pauker and Kassirer in 1980.[1] Imagine diagnostic testing as two separate thresholds, each denoted as 'I' (Fig. 1.1). The scale at the bottom of Fig. 1.1 denotes pre-test probability, which is the probability of the disease in question before any testing is employed. The threshold between 'don't test' and 'test' is known as the testing threshold; between 'test' and 'treat' is what is known as the test-treatment threshold. In this schema, treatment should be withheld if the pre-test probability of disease is smaller than the testing threshold and no testing should be performed. Treatment should be given without testing if the pre-test probability of disease is approximately equal to the test-treatment threshold. And then, when the pre-test probability lies between the testing and test-treatment thresholds, the test should be performed and the patient treated according to the test results. That is the theory; now let's make this more clinically relevant.

Sometimes disease is clinically apparent and we do not need confirmatory testing before proceeding with treatment. If you are evaluating a patient with an obvious cellulitis, you may choose to give antibiotics before initiating any testing. How about the evaluation of a 50-year-old male with chest pain who has large inferior 'tombstone' ST-segment elevations on his electrocardiogram consistent with acute myocardial infarction (AMI)? Cardiac markers are not likely to be very helpful in the acute management of this patient. This is another example where it is important to treat the patient first: give them

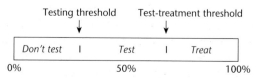

Figure 1.1 Pre-test probability of disease.

aspirin and beta-blockers, anticoagulate them, provide oxygen, and send them off to the cardiac catheterization laboratory if your hospital has one, or provide intravenous thrombolysis if cardiac catheterization is not readily available. Now imagine that the patient has a history of Marfan's syndrome and you think the patient is having an acute AMI, but you want to get a chest X-ray to make sure that they don't have an aortic dissection before you anticoagulate them. That might put you on the 'test' side of the line. If the test is positive for what may be a dissection, you won't give aspirin and anticoagulate; if it's negative, you will.

The scenario of the potential use for tissue plasminogen activator (tPA) in stroke patients frequently comes up in the ED. When a patient comes to the ED within the first 3 hours after the onset of their stroke symptoms, you rush to get a patient to the CT scanner. Why? The primary reason is to differentiate between ischemic and hemorrhagic stroke, which will make a major difference to whether or not the patient is even eligible to receive tPA.

Now imagine cases where you are below the testing threshold. You have a 32-year-old male with what appears to be musculoskeletal chest pain. Some would argue that the patient doesn't need any emergency tests at all if the patient is otherwise healthy and the physical examination is normal. Others might get a chest X-ray and an electrocardiogram to rule out occult things like pneumothorax and heart disease, while some others may even get a D-dimer to rule out pulmonary embolism. Which of these is the right way to manage the patient? Is there any evidence behind that decision or is it just physician's preference? In some patients, at the end of the ED evaluation you may still not have a definitive answer. Imagine you have a 45-year-old female with atypical chest pain and normal electrocardiogram and cardiac marker results, and your hospital does not perform stress testing from the ED. Does she need a hospital admission for rule out and a stress test?

The way that Pauker and Kassirer[1] designed the test-treatment thresholds almost 30 years ago did not account for the proliferation of 'confirmatory' diagnostic testing in hospitals. While the lower boundary of the testing threshold is certainly lower than it has ever been, the upper boundary has also increased as there are occasions when we are loathed to treat before testing, even when the diagnosis seems apparent. The reason for this is that Occam's razor does not often hold true in emergency medicine.

So what is Occam's razor? In the 14th century William of Occam stated that "plurality must not be posited without necessity," which has been interpreted to mean 'among competing hypotheses, favor the simplest one.'[2] When applied to test-treatment thresholds, what we find is that a patient with objective findings for what might seem like pneumonia (that is hypoxia, infiltrate, and a history of cough) is likely to have pneumonia and should be treated empirically as such, but may also have a pulmonary embolism. While finding parsimony of diagnosis is important, often the principle of test-treatment thresholds means that if you are above the test-treatment threshold then you should certainly treat, but also consider carrying out more tests, particularly in patients with objective signs of disease.

Think about how trauma surgeons practice. When the multi-injured trauma patient is seen, isn't their approach to test, test, test? If you are already injured and another part hurts, get a CT scan. Some order CT scans on patients where it doesn't even hurt; the thinking behind this approach is not illogical. When a patient has been in a major car accident and has a broken left femur and a broken left radius and mild abdominal tenderness, do they need more CT scans to rule out intra-abdominal injuries and intracranial injuries? Where Occam's razor dulls is in the situation when although the most parsi-monious diagnosis (just a radius and femur fracture) is possible, patients with multiple traumatic injuries tend to have not only the obvious ones, but also tend to have occult injuries too. This necessitates the diagnostic search for the occult intra-abdominal, intra-thoracic, and intra-cranial injuries in the patient with the obviously broken arm and leg.

When deciding on care plans, we develop our own risk tolerance based on our training, clinical expertise, and experiences, and on the local standard practice, and attitudes of the patient, family, or other physicians caring for the patient. Risk tolerance guides where we draw our own individual testing and test-treatment thresholds, and how much effort we put into searching for the occult. Risk tolerance refers to the post-test probability that we are com-fortable with, having excluded a disease or confirmed a disease. That is, risk tolerance is where we are comfortable setting our testing and test-treatment thresholds.

For example, let's say we are evaluating someone for a possible acute coronary syndrome. At the end of the ED stay after an electrocardiogram, chest X-ray, and evaluation of their cardiac marker levels, you calculate that they have a 2% risk of being sent home and having an unexpected event within 30 days. Is it OK to send them home with this level of risk? Isn't that the published rate for missed AMI? What if the risk is 1%, or 0.5%, or 0.1%?

How do you make the decision about when to order a test to just treat? How do you assign a pre-test probability? How do you apply test results to an individual patient? This is where research and the practice of evidence-based medicine (EBM) can influence medical practice by taking the best evidence from the literature about diagnostic testing or clinical decision rules and using that information to make an informed decision about how to care for patients. Chapters 2 and 3 provide an overview of the process of EBM and examples of its application to individual patients in the ED. Chapter 4 comprises a discussion of how we derive, validate, and study the impact of clinical decision rules in practice.

Understanding the evidence behind diagnostic testing and using clinical decision rules to decide not to test is at the core of emergency medicine practice. Think back to your last shift in the ED; how many tests did you order?

The purpose of this book is to demystify the evidence behind diagnostic testing and clinical decision rules in emergency care by going back and carefully evaluating the evidence behind our everyday decision making. This book is written to provide objective information on the evidence behind these questions and our opinion on how we manage our patients with that clinical problem given the best available evidence. Now, keep in mind that we are writing this from the perspective of academic emergency physicians. We work in an inner city ED with abundant (although not always quick) access to consultants, a state-of-the-art laboratory, and high-resolution imaging tests. Physicians in our practice also tend to have somewhat of a testing threshold, where patients often have testing done for minor symptoms. As you read this, realize that not all emergency medicine practice is the same and you should interpret the literature yourself in the context of your own clinical practice environment.

We have designed each chapter around clinical questions that come up in everyday emergency medicine practice. For each question, we present the objective data from published studies and then provide our 'expert' comment on how we use these tests in our practice. We try to provide insights into how we interpret the literature for each testing approach. Again, our comments should not necessarily be interpreted as the standard of care in emergency medicine. Standard of care is based on practice guidelines and local practice patterns. Instead, these chapters should serve as a forum or a basis for discussion for each clinical question. If you are a researcher, you can also think of this book as a roadmap to what is really 'known' or 'not known' with regard to diagnostic testing in emergency medicine, and what needs further study. Finally, rigorous and sound research often takes months to years to accomplish, and sometimes longer to publish. Therefore the discussions we present are likely to change as newer, larger, and more comprehensive studies are published, as new prediction or decision rules are validated and replicated, and as newer diagnostic technology is introduced.

References

1. Pauker, S.G. and Kassirer, J.P. (1980) The threshold approach to clinical decision making. *New England Journal of Medicine* **302**: 1109–1117.
2. Drachman, D.A. (2000) Occam's razor, geriatric syndromes, and the dizzy patient. *Annals of Internal Medicine* **132**: 403–404.

Chapter 2 **Evidence-Based Medicine: the Process**

The process that we use in this book has been termed evidence-based medicine (EBM). The first and most important question is "what is EBM?" EBM has been defined as "the conscientious, explicit and judicious use of current best evidence in making decisions about the care of patients".[1] The best way to describe EBM in the emergency department (ED) is a process by which we: (i) ask relevant clinical questions; (ii) go out and search for data; (iii) evaluate the data; and (iv) use that data in everyday clinical practice and apply it to the way that we manage individual patients. For this book, we use the process of EBM to answer important and relevant clinical questions that come up everyday while working in the ED regarding the use of diagnostic testing and clinical decision rules. Most of the questions we ask and attempt to answer in this book have to do with how to use, when to use, and how much to trust diagnostic testing and clinical decision rules, and then how to apply published knowledge to individual patients. EBM can also be used for other applications in emergency care outside of diagnostic testing, such as determining which treatment is best for an individual patient. However, in this book we will be focusing on diagnostic testing and clinical decision rules.

The purpose of this chapter is to go through the steps of EBM in detail and to discuss how to use EBM in the practice of emergency care with regard to diagnostic testing. The practice of EBM is a process that follows four simple steps, as shown in the list below.

Step 1: Formulate a clear question from a patient's problem. Does this patient need a test? Which test do they need? For example, does a patient with atypical chest pain who is otherwise low risk need a troponin test? You may ask

Evidence-Based Emergency Care: Diagnostic Testing and Clinical Decision Rules. By J.M. Pines and W.W. Everett. Published 2008 by Blackwell Publishing, ISBN: 978-14051-5400-0.

yourself, "how good is troponin I as a screening test for excluding acute coronary syndrome in ED patients?" Ask yourself, is this an answerable question?

Step 2: Search the literature for clinical articles that have addressed this question. Ideally, the sample will include ED patients with a similar complaint or disease process (i.e. patients with chest pain who are low risk for acute coronary syndrome where troponin has been studied). You might start by doing searches on patients with chest pain in the ED then narrow your search to include only articles that deal with the use of cardiac biomarkers.

Step 3: Read and critically appraise the articles for validity and applicability to the individual patient. That is, you can ask yourself "would the patient have met the inclusion criteria for this study?" or "Is this patient similar to patients who were included in the study?"

Step 4: Use the study findings and apply them to the care of an individual patient (i.e. does this patient need a troponin I test?) or to how you approach the use of cardiac troponins in the ED.

EBM problems are broken down into two categories: (i) general medical questions (i.e. what is the sensitivity of urine leukocyte esterase in diagnosing urinary tract infections?); and (ii) specific patient-based questions (i.e. in a 45-year-old female without risk factors, atypical chest pain, and nonspecific ECG changes, what is the value of a negative troponin?). In general, throughout this book we ask the former type of general medical questions, but we do give examples of the latter in the first three chapters. We recommend that you use our interpretation of the literature as a starting point, from which you can follow the same process to answer specific questions and hence apply your own interpretation of the literature to guide diagnostic plans.

The acronym 'PICO' has been used to define the four elements of an answerable question regarding a diagnostic test.[2] When referring to studies on diagnostic testing, PICO consists of the: (i) patient/population; (ii) investigation; (iii) comparison, i.e. what is the gold standard; and (iv) outcome of interest. In our prior example, P = women in their 40s without cardiac risk factors, I = troponin I measurement, C = cardiac catheterization or possible coronary angiogram, and O = identification of an intervenable coronary artery lesion or the presence of coronary artery disease (for risk stratification).

Once you have come up with a clinical question that is answerable then the search begins. For those of you who have access to online databases (such as MEDLINE), it is probably best to start there because you can enter specific search criteria and narrow your search as appropriate. Websites such as www.pubmed.com allow access to abstracts and some full text articles; sometimes hospitals and universities will allow a greater level of access to full-text articles through institutional memberships.

OK, you're logged on; what now? What you can do is either search by using a specific set of search criteria like 'troponin' and 'chest pain,' or you can use a more rigorous approach such as a using the Medical Subject Headings (MeSH) system. MeSH is a vocabulary that is used to index articles in MEDLINE/PubMed. It is probably a more consistent way to search because different terminology is sometimes used for the same topic. Just like what the British call the boot, the Americans call a trunk. These differences are even more common in medical terminology. For example, you may want to know about shortness of breath, but papers on this may describe shortness of breath in other ways, such as respiratory distress, dyspnea, or breathlessness. Another way to search PubMed is by using a 'clinical query,' which allows the user to search for specific clinical studies by diagnosis. Another common trick to use is to impose 'limits' on your search, which allows you to search for articles of a specific type, such as reviews, or to limit searches to specific age ranges, gender, publication dates, or language of publication. After finding the best evidence you can find on a clinical topic, you then need to do your own critical appraisal of the literature. Traditionally, assessment of the literature surrounding a clinical topic is good fodder for group discussion in either a conference or a residency journal club, but you can also go directly to the literature to answer important and relevant clinical questions yourself.

The assessment of studies involving diagnostic tests follows four critical steps,[3] which are detailed in the list below.

Step 1: Was there an independent, blind comparison with a reference standard (i.e. gold standard) for diagnosis? Examples of relevant gold standards in emergency medicine include surgical evaluation or biopsy results at laparotomy or laparoscopy for patients with appendicitis, cardiac catheterization results for patients with possible acute coronary syndrome, and pulmonary angiogram results for patients with potential pulmonary embolism. There may also be other ways to incompletely measure a gold standard, like the use of a negative chest CT followed by negative leg ultrasounds in patients with pulmonary embolism.

Step 2: Was the diagnostic test under question evaluated in the same population of patients as the patient in question? You can stratify this question by age, gender, location (i.e. were they ED patients?), or presenting symptoms (i.e. patients with chest pain). That is, when I read that the sensitivity for D-dimer is 95% in a meta-analysis, is my patient similar to the ones that were included in those studies?

Step 3: Did all patients have the reference standard test or follow-up, whereby you can be convinced that the test was either positive or negative? An example of this is if we only perform the gold standard test on patients with positive test results then this may skew the results of our assessment of sensitivity. For example, if we only do temporal artery biopsies on patients with positive erythrocyte sedimentation rates (ESRs) you may miss some patients who had a negative ESR and would have had a positive biopsy. This is called 'verification bias.'

Step 4: Has the test been validated in another independent group of patients? This is particularly concerning when the test is derived and validated in a specific population. For example, if a diagnostic test works well in Canada, does that mean it will have the same test characteristics in Boston?

Assessing studies on clinical decision rules is related but a little different and also involves four steps, which are detailed in the following list[4].

Step 1: Were the patients chosen in an unbiased fashion and do the study patients represent a wide spectrum of severity of disease? For example, did the enrollment criteria for the Canadian Head CT Rule include patients with minor bumps with a loss of consciousness through to major head injuries?

Step 2: Was there a blinded assessment of the gold standard for all patients? That is, did all patients who were enrolled in the study have CT scans?

Step 3: Was there an explicit and accurate interpretation of the predictor variables and the actual rule without knowledge of the outcome? Were the study forms filled out before the physicians had knowledge of the CT results? Was there an assessment of inter-rater reliability?

Step 4: Was follow-up obtained for 100% of patients who were enrolled? For patients who were discharged, did they follow them up to make sure that they did not have pain, any positive head CT scans, or poor outcome in a specific time period?

If you read a study or series of studies about a test or a clinical decision rule that does not meet the criteria detailed in either of the two lists shown above, you should be appropriately skeptical. However, in actual practice and as we found in writing this book, for many topics it is difficult to find literature that fulfills all of these specifications. In that case what we need to do is to interpret the literature whilst being aware of its weaknesses, and to do our best to apply the results to how we practice medicine. Certainly, for some tests, there may be a huge literature from which we can make strong recommendations (such as for D-dimer or the Ottawa Ankle Rules). For others, like using an ESR to rule out temporal arteritis, there may be no literature that meets all these requirements.

The next step is to use these findings and apply them to individual patients and thus integrate your understanding of the literature into clinical practice. Chapter 3 describes in detail the terms sensitivity, specificity, likelihood ratios, and Bayesian analysis, and discusses the mathematics behind the practical application of what we learn from studies to individual patients. By determination of a specific pre-test probability (or prevalence) of the disease in a particular patient, this can then help us to not only calculate a post-test probability but also to decide whether we need to perform the test at all.

The purpose of the process of diagnostic testing is not necessarily to reach 100% certainty; instead we are trying to reduce the level of uncertainty to allow us to optimize medical decision making. In order to move between test and test-treatment thresholds then we need to remember back to Chapter 1 and only order tests that ultimately change patient management and move us over a specific threshold.

There are potential pitfalls in the application of EBM to diagnostic testing and clinical decision rules. The first potential pitfall is in trying to describe the 'P' component (patient/population) without being too exclusive. Let's say we are trying to determine what the sensitivity of the troponin I test is for a 45-year-old woman with atypical chest pain and a non-diagnostic ECG. There is not likely to be any one specific study that describes troponin sensitivity in 45-year-old women with that exact description. On the other hand, if we are too vague in how we choose the 'P' component it can become similarly frustrating. For example, let's say we wanted to determine the test sensitivity for this patient using a study that includes patients of different ages with all sorts of complaints.

The 'I' component (investigation) is generally fairly straightforward, but for diagnostic testing clinicians need to be aware that there is sometimes poor standardization. We need to be aware of which test our laboratory uses. Does your hospital use the D-dimer enzyme-linked immunosorbant assay (ELISA) or immunoassay? The reason that this is important is because the sensitivities for the two tests are actually different. Therefore, the results for a published assay will not necessary be identical to those obtained from the assay used in your hospital; you should keep this in mind.

The 'C' component is the comparison. A comparison is typically a gold standard test for whatever you might be interested in studying. The gold standard is the most definitive test there is. For example, for appendicitis the gold standard would be a histologic diagnosis of inflammation of the appendix. In some studies, gold standard tests may not be ordered on all patients because often gold standard tests may have a high risk of complications (like pulmonary angiogram for pulmonary embolism). Another way that is not as good that researchers use for patients who have not had the gold standard is either a series of tests or some form of follow-up evaluation, such as a 14-day follow-up phone call for patients with potential C-spine fractures; if they are not having pain at 14-days, it is likely that they did not have a fracture.

The 'O' component is the outcome. Outcomes should be objective and clear. For example, was the patient alive at 30 days? Survival is an outcome that is difficult to dispute. Some outcomes are not ideal in the emergency medicine literature, such as whether a patient was admitted or not. Because some admission decisions can be subjective, you should be skeptical of studies that use subjective outcomes where there is the possibility of inter-rater variability in the key outcome.

Once a question has been framed using PICO, literature searching is also straightforward. Care should be given to use limit searches appropriately. For example, age limits should be set if you are studying children. However, when you are studying older adults, limiting it to an upper bound can sometimes result in the exclusion of important studies.

In conclusion, understanding the process of EBM can allow you to move from the general medical questions that we have attempted to answer in this book to the application of these principles to patient care in the ED. Understanding the pitfalls is important, as is sitting down and practicing clinical scenarios to see if you can make this process work for you.

References

1. Sackett, D.L., Rosenberg, W.M., Gray, J.A., Haynes, R.B. and Richardson, W.S. (1996) Evidence based medicine: what it is and what it isn't. *British Medical Journal* **312**: 71–72.
2. Sackett, D.L., Richardson, W.S., Rosenberg, W. and Haynes, R.B. (1998) *Evidence-Based Medicine: How to Practice and Teach EBM.* Churchill Livingstone, Oxford.
3. Jaeschke, R., Guyatt, G.H. and Sackett, D.L. (1994) How to use an article about a diagnostic test. A. Are the results of the study valid? *Journal of the American Medical Association* **271**: 389–391.
4. Richardson, W.S. and Detsky, A.S. (1995) How to use a clinical decision analysis. A. Are the results of the study valid? *Journal of the American Medical Association* **273**: 1292–1295.

Chapter 3 **The Epidemiology and Statistics of Diagnostic Testing**

Throughout much of this book, we will be referring to diagnostic test characteristics including sensitivity, specificity, negative predictive value, positive predictive value, and likelihood ratios. There are also references to common epidemiological terms such as incidence and prevalence. Terms that denote risk are odds and probability, and the odds ratio is commonly used in the literature to denote comparative risk among populations. Confidence intervals are also a frequently used but sometimes misunderstood concept. There is also the term 'spectrum bias' that is used in reference to diagnostic testing and the interpretation of studies about diagnostic testing. Another more complex statistic that we will describe because it is frequently used in diagnostic testing is the receiver operator curve (ROC). This chapter will provide explanations of the terms that we use in this book and will offer examples of how they can be used in clinical practice in the emergency department (ED).

The 2 × 2 table

Throughout this chapter and in other areas of this book we will be using the following 2 × 2 table format, which you may remember (and tried to forget) from your biostatistics class in medical school:

Evidence-Based Emergency Care: Diagnostic Testing and Clinical Decision Rules. By J.M. Pines and W.W. Everett. Published 2008 by Blackwell Publishing, ISBN: 978-14051-5400-0.

		Disease		
		+	−	Total
Test	+			
	−			
	Total			

In the top row of the table the 'disease' is listed and on the left-hand side of the table the 'test' is listed. Both 'disease' and 'test' are further broken down into '+', '−' and 'total'. For 'disease', a '+' means that the disease is present and a '−' means that the disease is absent; similarly for 'test' a '+' denotes a positive result and a '−' denotes a negative result.

Using information in these cells, all of the common test characteristics including sensitivity, specificity, positive predictive value, negative predictive value, and likelihood ratios can be calculated. We can also take a pre-test probability (i.e. the probability that a patient has a specific condition before a test is applied) of disease, apply known sensitivity and specificity, and hence calculate a post-test probability. These 2 × 2 tables can be very helpful in the ED if you know how to use them properly. A thorough understanding of them can allow you to apply 'real-time' evidence-based medicine (EBM). The way we do it is to first calculate a pre-test probability based on either a validated risk stratification tool or on our own clinical judgment. Accurately assigning a pre-test probability is both an art and a science. You have to think about the overall prevalence of disease—is it common or rare? Then you have to think about how prevalent the disease might be in the individual patient under question. Aside from certain widely studied disease like pulmonary embolism and acute coronary syndrome (ACS), it is often difficult to know whether the pre-test probability that you are assigning is correct. Often, you must make a guess, which seems rather arbitrary given the complex mathematics and calculations that ensue from this choice.

The next step is to apply a diagnostic test with known sensitivity and specificity. From that we can establish what the post-test probability is (i.e. the probability that a patient has a specific condition after the test results are known). Using a post-test probability, we can then decide how to proceed with the care of an individual patient. Now that is EBM in practice!

Sensitivity and specificity

Sensitivity refers to the ability of a test to detect a disease when it is actually present. A common acronym that has been used to remember sensitivity is 'PID' or positive in disease. In terms of the 2 × 2 table, sensitivity can be demonstrated as follows:

		Disease		
		+	−	Total
Test	+	85		
	−	15		
	Total	100		

In this example, of 100 people with a disease, 85 of them will have a positive test and 15 will have a negative test (also known as false negatives). The sensitivity of the test will therefore be 85/100 or 85%.

In contrast, **specificity** correctly identifies the absence of disease. That is, in people who do not have the disease, specificity denotes the percentage of those who will have a negative test. This can be easily remembered by the acronym 'NIH' or negative in health. In the 2 × 2 table, specificity can be demonstrated as follows:

		Disease		
		+	−	Total
Test	+		20	
	−		80	
	Total		100	

In this case, of the 100 people without disease, 80% will have negative test results while 20% of patients will have positive results (also known as false positives). The test specificity is therefore 80/100 or 80%.

Spectrum bias

Spectrum bias is common in diagnostic testing and occurs when there are differing sensitivities and specificities in different subpopulations. Subpopulations can correspond to either different severities of illness or some other factor that differentiates risk in patients. For example, in the case of subarachnoid hemorrhage computed tomography (CT) scan sensitivity will change over time, with the greatest degree of sensitivity seen soon after the onset of a sentinel headache and the lowest level of sensitivity 12–24 h after onset. Another example of spectrum bias is where test sensitivity will be variable at different clinical likelihoods of disease. Rapid strep tests are an example of spectrum bias where in patients with sore throats higher Centor scores (denoting a higher probability of a positive group A *Streptococcus* infection) means that the sensitivity of the tests will be higher.

Incidence and prevalence

The **prevalence** of disease is defined as the proportion of people who have a disease within a population at any one point of time. **Incidence** is related to prevalence but differs in that incidence refers to new cases of a disease over a certain period of time. For example, assuming that we have a healthy population of 1000 people on January 1, and by December 31, five had developed a specific disease, the disease incidence would be 5 per 1000 per year.

Using our 2 × 2 table, we can demonstrate the concept of prevalence in the following way:

		Disease		
		+	−	Total
Test	+			
	−			
	Total	100	100	200

Thus, of the total population of 200 people, 100 people have the disease (i.e. they are disease positive) and 100 people do not have the disease (i.e. they are disease negative). In this population, the overall prevalence is 100/200 or 50%. Sensitivity and specificity are independent of the prevalence of disease in the population as you can see from the following table:

		Disease		
		+	−	Total
Test	+	85	20	105
	−	15	80	95
	Total	100	100	200

That is to say, sensitivity and specificity do not change when the prevalence changes; instead, predictive values change—except for when there is spectrum bias.

Predictive values

Positive predictive value is the probability that the disease is present if the test is positive. This can be illustrated as:

		Disease		
		+	−	Total
	+	85	20	105
Test	−			
	Total			

In this case, of the 105 people with positive tests, 85 actually have the disease. Therefore, the positive predictive value is 85/105 or 81%.

The **negative predictive value** is the probability that the disease is absent if the test is negative, which is illustrated in the following 2 × 2 table:

		Disease		
		+	−	Total
	+			
Test	−	15	80	95
	Total			

Of the 95 people with negative tests, 80 do not have the disease. Therefore, the negative predictive value is 80/95 or 84%.

Integrating concepts

Another way to integrate sensitivity and specificity with predictive values is by using mnemonics. The mnemonics 'snout', or sensitivity (rule out), and 'spin', or specificity (rule in), have been proposed. When you want to rule something out (e.g. by deciding upon a clinical decision rule or a diagnostic

test for a low-risk patient), then the ideal test should have near perfect sensitivity. This will result in a correspondingly high negative predictive value (i.e.
the disease is ruled out). Conversely, when you are trying to rule something
in, ideal tests have near perfect specificity, which will correspond to a high
positive predictive value (i.e. the disease will be ruled in).

Using 2 × 2 tables: an example

In contrast to sensitivity and specificity, the positive and negative predictive
values do change with changing disease prevalence. For the moment, let's
assume that there is no spectrum bias. As an example you go to see a patient
and, based on your initial assessment, there is a high pre-test probability of
disease. Let's set the pre-test probability estimate at 80%. If we take the same
test characteristics that we had in the prior example, where sensitivity is 85%
and specificity is 80%, what happens to the predictive values?

First, we start with the disease prevalence (80%) where, in a hypothetical
population of 200 people, 160 have the disease and 40 do not.

		Disease		
		+	−	Total
	+			
Test	−			
	Total	160	40	200

We then add in the known sensitivity (85%) and specificity (80%). The
number of true positives will be 136, false positives 8, true negatives 32, and
false negatives 24:

		Disease		
		+	−	Total
	+	136	8	144
Test	−	24	32	56
	Total	160	40	200

Now, if we have a positive test in this population, the positive predictive
value would be 136/144 or 94% (which is higher than it would be if the prevalence was 50%) and the negative predictive value would be 32/56 or 57%

(which is lower than it would be if the prevalence was 50%). What tends to happen is that as your prevalence goes up, a positive test is *more* likely to be a true positive and a negative test is *less* likely to be a true negative.

So how does this work if the disease prevalence is low? Let's set a prevalence of 10%:

		Disease		
		+	−	Total
	+			
Test	−			
	Total	20	180	200

Now, if we apply the same test characteristics where sensitivity is 85% and specificity is 80%:

		Disease		
		+	−	Total
	+	17	36	53
Test	−	3	144	147
	Total	20	180	200

In this case, the positive predictive value is 17/53 or 32% (which is less than it was when the population prevalence was 50%) and the negative predictive value is 144/147 or 98% (which is higher than when the population prevalence was 50%). In this case, because the prevalence is low, a positive test is less likely to be a true positive and a negative test is more likely to be a true negative.

As a general principle, as your disease prevalence goes up, your positive predictive value increases. As your disease prevalence goes down, your negative predictive value increases. In other words, if you are worried about a patient and you think they are high risk for the disease, then if the test is positive it has a good chance of being a true positive. Conversely, if a patient is probably OK and you have ordered an imperfect test (like an electrocardiogram to rule out ACS in a 25 year old), which comes back normal, the likelihood that it is a true negative is very high.

Another way to think about prevalence is in terms of pre-test probability. After you see and evaluate a patient, the prevalence is equal to the pre-test probability for that individual patient. If you see 100 patients with the same presentation, what percentage will have the disease? Put another way, you can use the disease '+/−/total' boxes using pre-test probability to determine your predictive values for an individual patient.

Let's use an example of a specific patient to illustrate how we can use EBM at the bedside in emergency medicine. Imagine you are evaluating a 55-year-old female who presents with intermittent, sharp, right-sided chest pain and shortness of breath for one week. She has no traditional risk factors for pulmonary embolism or coronary artery disease. She has a normal physical examination except for tenderness to palpation over the right side of the chest. Vitals are within normal limits except for a heart rate of 110 beats per minute that is regular.

You are considering the diagnosis of pulmonary embolism in this patient and you want to determine the risk of them having this condition. So you pose your question, you search the literature and then you evaluate a study on the Wells criteria and decide to use it. According to the Wells criteria, you assign 1.5 points for a heart rate of ≥100 beats per minute based upon your clinical judgment. This places her in a 'low-risk' category. In addition, you assign her a pre-test probability of 3.6% based on the Wells criteria, which was the prevalence of pulmonary embolism in that category in the original study. While this is not likely to be her exact pre-test probability, you do agree that she is relatively low risk for pulmonary embolism.

Because she is low risk, you decide to order a D-dimer on her. You think back to the key questions: "what will I do if it's positive?" or "what if it's negative?" Let's go back to the 2 × 2 tables to see. You first start by entering her pre-test probability. Of every 100 patients you see that are identical to this one, approximately 7 in 200 will have the disease:

		Disease		
		+	−	Total
Test	+			
	−			
	Total	7	193	200

Now, let's look up the sensitivity and specificity for D-dimer. We found a review article in MEDLINE that shows that in a meta-analysis, D-dimer sensitivity was 94% and the specificity was 45%.[1] Conveniently, our hospital just so happens to use the same D-dimer assay as that used in this meta-analysis. Let's enter the numbers and see what we get:

		Disease		
		+	−	Total
Test	+	6	106	112
	−	1	87	88
	Total	7	193	200

Well, it's not perfect, but let's say for simplicity that D-dimer will pick up 6/7 (85%) of the patients with disease to make the numbers fit.

So our test is positive; what is the positive predictive value? We can calculate that this is 6/112 or 5%. This is not very good; with a positive D-dimer we have moved our pre-test probability from 3.6% to a post-test probability of 5.4%. This certainly does not push us over any treatment threshold. That is, we do not want to anticoagulate people who have a 5.4% chance of having the disease with heparin or enoxaparin (the treatment for pulmonary embolism) because of the potential side effects of those medications. What if the test is negative? Well, then our negative predictive value is 87/88 or 98.9%. That's a pretty good negative predictive value. So, given a negative test, we have moved from a pre-test probability of 3.6% to a post-test probability of 1.2%. With a post-test probability of 1.2%, it may be reasonable to say that a diagnosis has been mostly excluded. As we can see from this example, D-dimer is a good rule-out test because the sensitivity is high and the specificity is poor. Remember: 'snout'.

Odds, probability, and the odds ratio

We will be using two related terms that denote risk in this book: odds and probability. People often use odds and probability interchangeably, but odds and probability actually mean different things. Probability makes more intuitive sense than odds in terms of how physicians see the world, but an odds ratio is often used in statistics to represent the likelihood that when comparing two groups, one will have the outcome in question.

Let's start with probability because this is the easiest to understand. The probability is the expected number over the total number. An easy example is to use six-sided dice. The probability of rolling a six on any individual roll is 1/6 or 16.7%. Using a hypothetical clinical example, the probability that a 50-year-old male who has risk factors for coronary disease, acute chest pain, and new electrocardiographic changes is having an ACS is high (let's say 80% as an estimate). That means, out of 100 identical patients, 80 of them will have ACS.

Odds are related but different. Odds are the ratio of the probability of occurrence to non-occurrence. Using the same example, the odds that you will roll a six is 1:5; while the odds that the 50-year-old male will have ACS is 4:1. You can convert odds to probabilities using the following formulas:

Odds = probability/(1 − probability)
Probability = odds/(1 + odds)

An odds ratio is a measure of the size of the difference between odds and is commonly used in the medical literature to denote risk. It is defined as a ratio of the odds of an event or outcome in one group to the odds of an event or outcome in another group. These groups are traditionally dichotomous classifications, like older people (≥65 years old) versus younger people (<65 years old), or men versus women. It can also be the difference between a treatment group and a control group. When the odds ratio is equal to 1, this indicates that the event or outcome is equally likely in both groups. When it is greater than 1, the condition or outcome is more likely in the first group. Finally, when it is less than 1, it is less likely in the first group. In an odds ratio, p is the probability of the outcome in group 1 and q is the probability of the outcome in group 2. As mentioned above, we can use the formula for odds to calculate an odds ratio in terms of probabilities:

Odds ratio = [p/(1 − p)]/[q(1 − q)]

As a clinical example, suppose that we have a sample of 100 male and 100 female ED patients with acute chest pain. This is only a theoretical example to demonstrate how to calculate an odds ratio and is not based on any studies. Of the 100 patients, 20 males and 10 females will have a serious cause for their pain. Thus the odds of a male having a serious cause for this pain are 20 to 80 or 1:4 while the odds of a female having a serious cause for her pain are 10 to 90 or 1:9. Using the above formula, we can calculate the odds ratio:

Odds ratio = [(0.20)/(1 − 0.20)]/[0.10/(1 − 0.10)] = 2.25

This calculation can be interpreted to mean that men have 2.25 times higher odds of have a serious cause for their chest pain than women. This also illustrates how an odds ratio can be larger than the difference in probability. While men are twice as likely to have a serious cause for their chest pain (in terms of probability), the odds ratio is higher (2.25).

Likelihood ratios

Likelihood ratios are a different way of interpreting sensitivity and specificity and provide a direct estimate of how much a test result (positive or negative) will change the odds of having a disease. The likelihood ratio for a positive result (LR+) tells you how much the odds of the disease increase when a test is positive. The likelihood ratio for a negative result (LR–) tells you how much the odds of the disease decrease when a test is negative.

In order to use likelihood ratios, you need to specify the pre-test odds. The pre-test odds are the likelihood that the patient would have a specific disease prior to any testing. Pre-test odds are related to the prevalence of disease and may be adjusted upwards or downwards depending on the characteristics of your overall patient pool (i.e. is the disease likely in your community) or of the individual patient (i.e. is the disease likely in the individual patient). To calculate likelihood ratios you can use the following formulas:

$$\text{LR+} = \text{sensitivity}/(1 - \text{specificity})$$
$$\text{LR–} = 1 - \text{sensitivity}/\text{specificity}$$
$$\text{Odds}_{post} = \text{odds}_{pre} \times \text{LR+} \text{ (a positive test)}$$
$$\text{Odds}_{post} = \text{odds}_{pre} \times \text{LR–} \text{ (a negative test)}$$

As a general rule of thumb, likelihood ratios greater than 10 or less than 0.1 generate sizeable changes in post-test disease probability, while likelihood ratios of 0.5–2 have little effect. It is also possible to use likelihood ratios when considering a sequence of independent tests (for example, an electrocardiogram followed by troponin I testing for potential ACS). Likelihood ratios can also be multiplied in series.

Using odds, probabilities and likelihood ratios: an example

The best way to describe odds, probabilities and likelihood ratios are by using a clinical example. Using D-dimer as an example, let's assume that the sensitivity is 94% and the specificity is 45%. We can calculate the LR+ to be 1.71 by the calculation $(0.94)/(1 - 0.45)$, and the LR– to be 0.13 from the calculation $(1 - 0.94)/(0.45)$.

OK, so let's go through the maths, starting with a pre-test probability of 10%. The first step is to convert that to an odds: $0.10/(1 - 0.10) = 0.1111$. So our pre-test odds value is 0.1111. If we want to apply likelihood ratios, we need to know our test results. If the test is positive, then given a LR+ of 1.71 we can calculate the post-test odds: $1.71 \times 0.1111 = 0.1899$. If the test is negative, we can apply a LR– of 0.13. So given a negative test result the post-test odds are $0.13 \times 0.1111 = 0.0144$. Now, we need to convert these back to probability values. An odds of 0.1899 is equal to a probability of $0.1899/(1 + 0.1899) = 16.0\%$. An odds of 0.0144 is equal to a probability of $0.0144/(1 + 0.0144) = 1.4\%$.

So let's put this into English. Given a pre-test probability of 10%, if you have a positive D-dimer your post-test probability is 16%. In this case, your post-test probability is also equal to your positive predictive value. If you have a negative test, your post-test probability is 1.4%. Another way of expressing a post-test probability when there is a negative test result is as a negative predictive value. In this case, your negative predictive value is 1 − post-test probability = (1 − 0.014) or 98.6%.

An even simpler way to work from a pre-test probability, modified by a likelihood ratio, to a post-test probability is to use a likelihood ratio nomogram (Fig. 3.1). Using a ruler, start from the pre-test probability in the left-hand

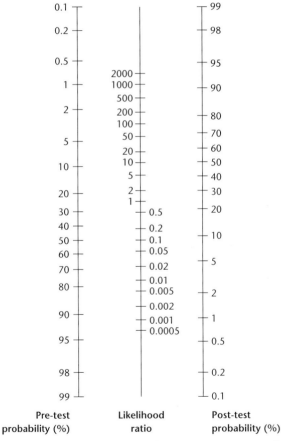

Figure 3.1 Likelihood ratio nomogram. To use the nomogram a pre-test probability is selected from the left-hand column and a line is drawn to the likelihood ratio (derived from the literature). Extending the line out to the right-hand column yields a post-test probability.

column and intersect the likelihood ratio value in the middle column. Extending the straight line from those two points out to the right-hand column results in the new post-test probability.

Bayes' theorem

To make things even more complicated, in order to calculate a post-test probability given a pre-test probability and known sensitivity and specificity, you can use Bayes' theorem and do it all in one step.

In the case of a positive test, you can calculate your post-test probability (or your positive predictive value) using the following formula:

Post-test probability
= (pre-test probability × sensitivity)/[(pre-test probability × sensitivity)
  + (1 − pre-test probability) × (1 − specificity)]

In the case of a negative test, you can calculate your post-test probability (i.e. 1 − negative predictive value) using the following formula:

Post-test probability
= (1 − pre-test probability) × specificity/{[(1 − pre-test probability) ×
  specificity] + [pre-test probability × (1 − sensitivity)]}

Let's go back to Chapter 1, when we mentioned the 83-year-old female with shortness of breath, chest pain, a history of pulmonary embolism, and a negative D-dimer. Given that her pre-test probability for pulmonary embolism is let's say 85%, we can calculate our post-test probability (and also our negative predictive value) using Bayes' theorem:

Post-test probability
= (1 − 0.85) × 0.45/{[(1 − 0.85) × 0.45] + [0.85 × (1 − 0.94)]}

This gives us a post-test probability of 61.3% and a negative predictive value of 1 − 0.613, or 38.7%. Given that her chance of pulmonary embolism is 61.3% after a negative test result, we have not safely ruled out pulmonary embolism. Therefore, she needs further testing such as chest CT or V/Q scans, or possibly even a pulmonary angiogram. Given that the pre-test probability was so high, you could make an argument to just treat her. But, given that anticoagulation is not without potential adverse effects, if you can order a confirmatory test then it is probably reasonable to do so.

So should we have ordered a D-dimer in the first place? The answer is probably not. In the case of a negative test, it did not help us because it did not move us over the test-treatment threshold.

Confidence intervals

Throughout this book we make reference to confidence intervals (CI). These are commonly used in statistics to give an estimated range of values that is likely to include an unknown population parameter (like an odds ratio or a population mean). As an easy example, let's say we are trying to estimate the average age of everyone living in a county of 50 000 people. In order to do this, we randomly select 100 houses and go door to door to find out what the ages are of everyone living at each house. This gives us a total sample of 322 people and we find that the average age is 32 years old. But how certain are we that 32 is the real average for the population? Instead of saying that 32 is the average, what we can do is give CI values. So we plug our numbers into our statistics program and what we find is that the average is indeed 32, but the 95% CI is 26–42. What we can say is that we are 95% sure that whatever the real value is (if we sampled all 50 000), it lies between 26 and 42 years old. Intervals are usually reported with 95% confidence, but if we want to be really sure we can report wider CI, such as 99%.

Let's use a clinical example. Like before, we want to know what the odds are for a male having a serious cause for chest pain compared to a female. What we would do is to go out and collect sample data to answer the question by studying males and females with chest pain and estimating the odds ratio based on the sample data. If we were to calculate an odds ratio of 2.25 with a 95% CI of 1.5–3.5, then what we can say is that we are 95% confident that the real difference between men and women falls between 1.5 and 3.5. Since it is greater than one, we can say that men are at higher risk of their chest pain being due to a serious cause than women.

Confidence interval width gives an indication of how uncertain we are about this unknown parameter. For example if we reported an odds ratio of 2.25 (95% CI 2.0–2.5), we could be fairly confident in our estimate. However, if we reported an odds ratio of 2.25 (95% CI 0.25–10.0), we would be less confident. A wide interval indicates that nothing very definite can be said about that particular parameter. As a rule of thumb, a parameter estimate with a small CI is more reliable than a result with a large CI.

Receiver operator characteristic (ROC) curves

Determination of sensitivity and specificity for a specific diagnostic test depends on the value that we define as an abnormal test. The threshold value that we set for an abnormal test will determine the number of true positives, true negatives, false positives and false negatives. For example, if we say an abnormal D-dimer test is at a specific threshold, let's say 500 ng/dL, then if we

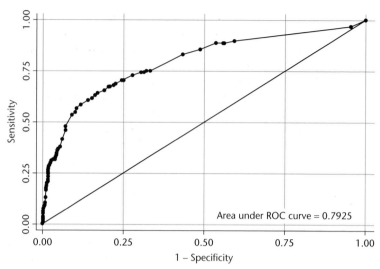

Figure 3.2 Receiver operator characteristic (ROC) curve.

were to set the cutoff at a higher level, let's say 2000 ng/dL, the number of both true positives and false negatives would increase. The purpose of ROC curves is to find the test cutoff that maximizes both sensitivity and specificity so that tests can be used and interpreted in clinically meaningful ways. Fig. 3.2 shows a typical ROC curve.

ROC curves are a way to plot test sensitivity and specificity at different values for thresholds that define positive and negative tests. Traditionally an ROC curve is a plot of the true positive rate (sensitivity) compared with the false positive rate (1 − specificity). The accuracy of a test is dependent on how well the test separates the group being tested into those with and without the disease. Test accuracy can be measured by the area under the ROC curve. If the area is equal to 1, then the test is perfect. An area of 0.5 is a worthless test. Table 3.1 provides a rough guide to classifying the accuracy of a diagnostic test using the area under the ROC curve.

Table 3.1 Determining the accuracy of a diagnostic test using the area under the ROC curve

Value	Accuracy
0.90–1.00	Excellent
0.80–0.90	Good
0.70–0.80	Fair
0.60–0.70	Poor

Another way of describing the area under the ROC curve is as test discrimination. It measures the ability of a test to correctly classify those with and without disease. Imagine a situation where we have two sets of patients, one with occult bacteremia and one without. If we were to randomly pick one patient from the group with bacteremia and one from the group without bacteremia and get white blood cell (WBC) counts for both, we should find that the patient with the highest WBC level is from the group with occult bacteremia. The area under the ROC curve is the percentage of randomly drawn pairs for which this is true (i.e. the test correctly classifies the two patients in the random pair). We will make reference to studies that use ROC curves throughout this book.

In conclusion, learning how to use diagnostic test characteristics (sensitivity, specificity, predictive values, and likelihood ratios), determine appropriate cutoffs and the accuracy of tests (ROC curves), report results (odds ratios and CIs), and understand the inherent bias in diagnostic testing (spectrum bias) can be helpful in the practice of EBM in the ED. An understanding of both the power and limitations of testing can aid in diagnosis and medical decision making.

Reference

1. Brown, M.D., Rowe, B.H., Reeves, M.J., *et al.* (2002) The accuracy of the enzyme-linked immunosorbent assay D-dimer test in the diagnosis of pulmonary embolism: a meta-analysis. *Annals of Emergency Medicine* **40**: 133–144.

Chapter 4 **Clinical Decision Rules**

Clinical decision rules are practical tools that are intended to assist us in deciding whether a diagnostic test is needed or what the likelihood is for the presence or absence of a particular disease or condition. They are designed to be simple and to provide a practical decision-making guide to differentiate patients who require testing or treatment from those who do not. Clinical decision rules typically include at least three elements from the patient's history, physical examination, and simple ancillary tests that can guide us at the bedside in the emergency department (ED) or in the office.[1] Decision rules are derived using a series of research studies on a specific clinical question. They must then be validated and tested in a different population. Each step in the derivation, validation, and external testing of a decision rule involves specific study designs and statistical analyses. At each stage in the development process, aspects of exactly how the study was conducted (i.e. patient population tested, specific outcomes) have an impact on how the rule should be interpreted and used in clinical practice. In this chapter we describe the steps researchers take to derive (generate) clinical decision rules and validate them (show that they work).

A decision rule is derived from a specific research question. When related to diagnostic testing, it traditionally starts with a question like: "XYZ is a disease that we often suspect but has a low positive testing rate. Is there a way to clinically differentiate cases with negative tests when there is a risk for XYZ, so that XYZ can be ruled out clinically without ordering any tests?" 'XYZ' may refer to common diseases that we want to exclude but which have a low prevalence of positives; for example intracranial bleeds, C-spine fractures, and knee and ankle fractures. How specific the clinical question may be suggests that there are limits to when a clinical decision rule can and should be used. For instance, consider the inclusion

Evidence-Based Emergency Care: Diagnostic Testing and Clinical Decision Rules. By J.M. Pines and W.W. Everett. Published 2008 by Blackwell Publishing, ISBN: 978-14051-5400-0.

criteria for a rule. If the derivation and validation of a decision rule regarding whether a blunt trauma patient should get a noncontrast head computed tomography (CT) scan to rule out intracranial pathology only included adult patients over the age of 18 years, the results may not be applied to similarly injured pediatric patients unless it was validated in that specific population.

Decision rules are intended to include elements of the patient's history, physical examination, or diagnostic tests that are reproducible and straightforward. Elements of clinical decision rules are also ideally binary (i.e. yes/no) or at least discrete with unambiguous options. We want to eliminate subjectivity as much as possible and maximize inter-rater reliability. This means that when two separate people assess an element of a rule, they have a high chance of agreeing on the results of that element. For example, few would argue that about a patient being 72 years old if the criterion was 'is the patient 65 and older?' it is likely that there would be perfect agreement between two individuals assessing this element. However, when we start using physical examination findings in a rule, such as does the patient have point tenderness over either malleolus of the ankle, then there is a greater chance for disagreement. This becomes further muddied when we try to use more subjective findings such as, is there rebound or guarding on an abdominal examination where clinicians may have a high likelihood of obtaining different results. Clinical decision rules also frequently do not take into context other intangible elements of the clinical setting. That is to say, clinical decision rules are not perfect. In the Canadian Head CT rule, a rule that determines whether or not patients require head CT scans after blunt head trauma, one of the elements includes a failure to reach a Glasgow Coma Scale (GCS) of 15 within 2 hours. If you are monitoring a patient who has the highest possible GCS but who starts to behave strangely 30 minutes after a blunt head trauma, you probably should not wait the 2 hours to see whether she normalizes. Rather, you should consider ordering a head CT early. Clinical decision rules often guide whether the likelihood of a disease is low enough to warrant the test. However, they are not necessarily binding. Even though clinical decision rules are designed to be 100% sensitive in theory, when tested in real-life practice they are almost always less than 100% sensitive. Clinical experience and gestalt are valuable assets in emergency medicine but are part of the intangible components that cannot be incorporated into clinical decision rules.

Over the past 15 years many decision rules have been introduced. The most notable and likely the most widely known are the sets of rules known as the Ottawa rules (the knee rules and ankle rules). Dr. Ian Stiell and his research colleagues in Ottawa, Canada have made a career of taking common clinical conditions where testing is frequently employed and positive tests are relatively rare, and trying to figure out who needs tests and who doesn't. By asking very simple and straightforward questions, Dr. Stiell's research has aimed to reduce unnecessary testing on patients by deriving decision rules to identify low risk patients who don't need tests. The other benefits of eliminating unnecessary testing using clinical decision rules include: (i) reductions of time in the ED for the patients; (ii) reduced exposure to radiation (for imaging); and (iii) reduced costs to both patients and the health care system overall.

The clinical decision rule development process

A first step in creating a rule is to consider a clinical situation that is common enough to warrant a decision rule. Is there a discrete and finite clinical question? For instance, does every patient with ankle pain need an X-ray? How frequently are tests positive? Ankle injuries are common and widespread complaints presenting to EDs around the world and ankle X-rays are frequently negative. Therefore, a rule that can identify low risk criteria to reduce unnecessary ankle radiography would be clinically helpful. So do we need a decision rule for patients with ankle pain? The clinical question is, "is there a fractured bone or not?" The practical question becomes, "is an X-ray needed?"

How do you go about creating a decision rule? The rest of this chapter will summarize the approach by describing the essential steps that researchers must undertake to develop a rule that is useful in practice. Several nicely written articles describing and discussing the methods for these components are available for those of you who want additional details.[1–5] As readers of the medical literature, developing a working understanding of each of these steps is important to determine, if you should use any specific decision rule for your patients.

The first step is **defining the outcome**. The outcome should be explicitly described and clinically relevant to the condition under study. For example, is there a fracture of either malleolus of the ankle? Does the patient have an acute appendicitis or a cervical spine fracture? All of these are discrete conditions with a binary yes or no answer. In describing the condition or test being examined, researchers also must define the patient population for the rule. Defining the outcome and the appropriate target patient population are essential because this determines the patient population to whom the rule can be applied.

Next, what are the most relevant and logical factors that might be used to predict an outcome or diagnosis? It is from the initial pool of **predictor**

variables that the final decision rule is derived. The predictor variables usually include demographic factors, medical history, circumstances surrounding the patient's injury (mechanism of injury, timing), results of the physical examination, and sometimes blood test results, electrocardiogram findings, or results of imaging studies. Accurately and consistently determining the presence of the predictor variables is the key to determining which variables should be ultimately included in the decision rule. Both the intraobserver agreement (i.e. repeated measurements by the same clinician) and interobserver agreement (i.e. measurements by different clinicians) should be high for inclusion in a decision rule. In terms of statistical measurement, researchers need to show that the predictor variables they are considering have sufficiently **high reproducibility**, in the form of kappa statistic (κ). A κ statistic is a number from 0 to 1, where 0 indicates no agreement and 1 indicates perfect agreement. Variables that are too subjective and have low κ values (<0.6) should not be included in the decision rule.

If the goal is to reliably exclude a fracture based on the history and physical findings for a patient with ankle pain, the predictor variables should be determined before knowledge of the X-ray results. Similarly, the X-ray results should not be interpreted solely on the basis of the history and physical examination findings. **Blinded assessment** of the predictor variables and outcomes from the imaging study ensures there is no observer or ascertainment bias in terms of the validity of the findings. For instance, let's say we have examined a patient and know there is point tenderness over the medial malleolus. We may review an X-ray more carefully in the area of concern looking for a fracture in that specific area, and may be more likely to call any irregularity a fracture. This is in contrast to a radiologist who is reading a similar X-ray without prior knowledge of the physical examination, and who concludes that there is no fracture present.

The **derivation phase** of a decision rule is a process of collecting the data in a standardized way, including the predictor variables, assessing the reliability of those data, and determining the outcome(s) being studied (in the ankle example the outcome is fracture). Researchers then use statistical methods to distill the predictor variables down to those that are the most predictive of the outcome. The two most common methods are recursive partitioning and logistic regression analysis. The former takes patients and divides them sequentially into groups with a particular outcome. Subsets of patients with that particular outcome are created based upon common predictor variables associated with the outcomes. Logistic regression analysis generates a model that predicts the outcome—which has to be binary (fracture or no fracture) —by using the best statistical combination of predictor variables. Functionally, this type of analysis creates odds of the outcome event based on the

Table 4.1 An example of the presentation of validation study results

	Outcome event (+)	Outcome event (−)
Clinical decision rule (+)	a	b
Clinical decision rule (−)	c	d

presence or absence of the predictor variables. The end result of both methods is a set of best predictor variables that comprise the decision rule.

The next phase following the derivation stage is the **validation phase**. During the validation phase the actual decision rule is applied to the patients for which they are intended and, in a blinded fashion, the outcomes are determined. The elements of the decision rule are assessed and recorded in a blinded format separate from the determination of the ultimate clinical outcome. The researchers then compare the performance of the decision rule with the outcome.

Validation usually takes the form of a 2 × 2 table, similar to the ones we saw in Chapter 2 (see Table 4.1) showing the results of the rule (rule positive or rule negative) compared to the outcome of the study (e.g. X-ray positive or X-ray negative). The results of the validation study should be clearly presented. When arranged in this format we can then calculate the sensitivity and specificity for a rule.

Sensitivity and specificity are performance characteristics of the rule or test being examined and are not influenced by the prevalence of the outcome event. Both positive and negative predictive values, on the other hand, change with the prevalence of the disease or outcome being studied, and therefore can and will change when the decision rule is applied to different populations or different settings. Statistical confidence in the results of the test performance should also be explicitly shown, usually in the format of 95% confidence intervals.

Some studies combine data collection for the derivation and validation phases in order to streamline the process. In these studies roughly half of the patient data is used to derive the best predictor variables for creating a decision rule. The remaining patient data is then used to validate the decision rule. This is perfectly acceptable so long as the patient sets are kept separate and distinct for each phase.

Issues of usability and practicality for the final rule need to be taken into account. The ease of use of a decision rule will be linked to its acceptance and use in clinical practice. Therefore, rules that have too many elements, or that are complicated to interpret or apply, or that have vague or subjective variables are less likely to be widely accepted.

The final steps in the decision rule evolution are assessing the impact and cost effectiveness of the rule in actual clinical practice. Reports of the impact of a decision rule are described in implementation studies. They reveal if the use of the rule results in changes in clinical practice and behavior patterns. Once effectiveness can be demonstrated, the economic effect can then be assessed. Demonstrating conservation of resources, health savings, increased efficiency, or, better still, all of these, can determine the success or failure of a decision rule.

The process from concept to final decision rule often takes several years to complete. The derivation and validation phases are often published separately. Implementation and cost-effectiveness studies for a clinical decision rule add additional years to a rule's long road to acceptance and use in clinical practice. Indeed, few decision rules have undergone these latter steps of testing. There is often a temptation to want to apply the results of a derivation study for a promising new decision rule based on the derivation study alone. We want to state explicitly that this should not be done, no matter how good the results appear to be. The initial validation and derivation studies often employ highly trained research personnel to record and elicit the data used in these studies and are, in effect, efficacy studies. That is, under ideal clinical research terms and settings can a rule be created and applied? This is different and distinct from effectiveness studies that examine how the rule works under regular routine clinical situations that are not study settings. A promising new decision rule should be examined critically and with caution. We should be sure to wait for external validation studies that replicate the findings in new or different setting from the initial sets of derivation/validation studies by different clinical researchers before incorporating a new decision rule into practice.

Unfortunately, few of the chapters in this book have a nice series of derivation, validation, implementation, and cost-effectiveness studies to describe and discuss. Instead many of the common clinical questions have only been partially evaluated or are in the formative stages of evaluation. Our hopes are that future studies will fill in the gaps that we point out; or, better still, that our discussions could fuel new exploration for clinically relevant questions with new, innovative decisions rules.

References

1. Laupacis, A., Sekar, N. and Stiell, I.G. (1977) Clinical prediction rules: a review and suggested modifications of methodological standards. *Journal of the American Medical Association* **277**(6): 488–494.

2. Randolph, A.G., Guyatt, G.H., Calvin, J.E., Doig, G. and Scott, R.W. (1998) Understanding articles describing clinical prediction tools. *Critical Care Medical* **26**(9): 1603–1612.
3. Stiell, I.G. and Wells, G.A. (1999) Methodological standards for the development of clinical decision rules in emergency medicine. *Annals of Emergency Medicine* **33**(4): 437–447.
4. McGinn, T.G., Guyatt, G.H., Wyer, P.C., Naylor, C.D., Stiell, I.G. and Richardson, W.S. (2000) Users' guide to the medical literature XXII: how to use articles about clinical decision rules. Evidence-Based Medicine Working Group. *Journal of the American Medical Association* **284**(1): 79–84.
5. Reilly, B.M. and Evans, A.T. (2006) Translating clinical research into clinical practice: impact of using prediction to make decisions. *Annals of Internal Medicine* **144**(3): 201–209.

SECTION 2
Traumatic Injuries

Chapter 5 **Cervical Spine Fractures**

Highlights

- The prevalence of cervical spine injuries from blunt trauma is low at around 1–2%.
- Applying either of the clinical decision rules for bluntly injured patients [Canadian C-spine rule (CCR) or the National Emergency X-Radiography Utilization Study (NEXUS) low-risk criteria (NLC)] helps identify low-risk patients in the emergency department (ED) for whom neck radiography can be deferred.
- Computed tomography (CT) imaging of the cervical spine is highly sensitive compared to plain film imaging, but should be reserved for selected patients at high risk of cervical spine injury.

Background

More than 14 million patients undergo radiographic imaging of the cervical spine each year in the US, with a clinically significant spine or cord injury found in less than 2% of all cases. As a result, many patients without injuries undergo negative radiographic imaging. The development of sensitive clinical decision rules to help clinicians identify patients that are at extremely low risk of a cervical spine injury has been helpful in reducing unnecessary imaging.

Two rules have been developed that use accepted clinical decision rule methodology: the NLC, and the CCR.[1,2] Each rule has been derived and validated in large and diverse populations of ED patients with very high sensitivity and negative predictive values.

There are also multiple radiographic modalities that are available to study the cervical spine including plain films (Fig. 5.1), computed tomography

Evidence-Based Emergency Care: Diagnostic Testing and Clinical Decision Rules. By J.M. Pines and W.W. Everett. Published 2008 by Blackwell Publishing, ISBN: 978-14051-5400-0.

(CT) scans (Fig. 5.2), and magnetic resonance imaging (MRI). While CT and MRI are more sensitive and are definitive tests, plain films are more widely available. Plain films also involve less radiation than CT scans. However, sometimes plain films are inadequate because of poor patient positioning and/or patient body habitus. When the lateral view does not have an adequate view of the C7–T1 space, repeat films with special views (i.e. swimmer's view) are often necessary. Instead of repeat films, physicians sometimes choose to perform CT scans on patients with inadequate X-rays, which further increases the radiation dose. MRI provides additional information over the CT scan in that it can identify ligamentous injuries.

Clinical question one

"Can a stable patient with blunt trauma be safely evaluated and the cervical spine cleared without undergoing radiographic imaging of the cervical spine?"
For the three highest quality studies available, a generally accepted definition of cervical spine injury included any fracture or ligamentous injury of the cervical spine. Each study also included an accepted list of acute fractures that are clinically stable and do not commonly result in surgical or other intervention. These clinically insignificant fractures include spinous process fractures, simple wedge fractures without loss of 25% or more of vertebral body height, isolated avulsion fractures without accompanying ligamentous injury, type 1 odontoid fractures, end plate fractures, fractures of osteophytes, trabecular bone injury, and transverse process fractures. For the purposes of rule derivation, these were not considered positive outcomes.

The NEXUS group formulated a clinical decision rule that included five elements:
- the absence of tenderness at the posterior midline of cervical spine;
- the absence of a focal neurologic deficit;
- a normal level of alertness;
- no evidence of intoxication; and
- the absence of clinically apparent pain that would distract a patient from the pain of a cervical injury.

The NLC were assessed as present, absent, or unable to be assessed. Whenever a component of the NLC was unassessable, the patient was considered not to have met that criterion. Patients that met all five criteria were considered to be at low risk for clinically significant cervical spine injury. Because they were low risk, NEXUS rules were designed such that these patients would not require imaging of the cervical spine in the ED.

The initial study for the NLC was a prospective observational study at 21 US medical centers that tested the hypothesis that blunt trauma patients who met all of the criteria would have an extremely low probability of cervical spine injury. All patients that underwent imaging of the cervical spine were included, except those that had a penetrating trauma or that required imaging of the cervical spine for a reason unrelated to trauma. Patients underwent the standard three-view imaging of the C-spine (lateral, anteroposterior, and open mouth views) or advanced imaging (CT, MRI). The NLC were applied in 34 069 patients and the incidence of radiographically documented cervical

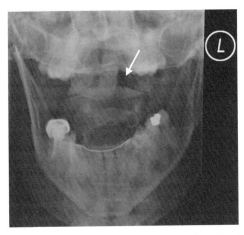

Figure 5.1 Open mouth odontoid cervical spine X-ray showing widening of the lateral pillar (arrow) of the first cervical vertebra, consistent with an acute fracture.

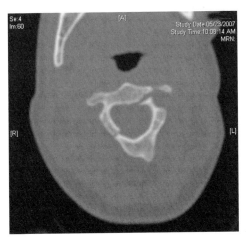

Figure 5.2 A second vertebral fracture is demonstrated on the cervical spine computed tomography scan.

Table 5.1 NEXUS low-risk criteria (NLC): study results and test performance from Hoffman *et al.*[1]

Assessment result for any cervical injury	Radiographically documented injury			Decision rule performance	
	Injury	No injury	Total		95% CI
Decision rule positive	810	28 950	29 760	Sensitivity 99.0%	98.0–99.6
				Specificity 12.9%	12.8–13
Decision rule negative	8	4 301	4 309	NPV 99.8%	99.6–100
				PPV 2.7%	2.6–2.8
Total	818	33 251	34 069		
Clinically significant cervical injury	Injury	No injury	Total		
Decision rule positive	576	29 184	29 760	Sensitivity 99.6%	98.6–100
				Specificity 12.9%	12.8–13
Decision rule negative	2	4 307	4 309	NPV 99.9%	99.8–100
				PPV 1.9%	1.8–2.0
Total	578	33 491	34 069		

NPV, negative predictive value; PPV, positive predictive value.

spine injury was 2.4%. Table 5.1 shows the results of the study and the performance of the NLC.

The criteria from this study missed a total of eight patients with documented cervical spine injuries. Only two of those injuries were clinically significant, and neither required surgical intervention or had any long-term clinical consequences. With 99.6% sensitivity and a 99.9% negative predictive value, it was felt that the patients from this large multicenter study met all of the criteria and could safely be considered as extremely low risk for cervical spine injury.

In a similar study performed at approximately the same time in Canada, Stiell and colleagues created the CCR. This decision rule was first published as a derivation study in 2001,[2] with the goal being to develop a prediction rule with extremely high sensitivity for detecting acute cervical spine injuries in stable ED patients with blunt trauma. The authors conducted a prospective cohort study in 10 Canadian EDs and derived the clinical and historical factors surrounding the injury that would optimize detection of a cervical spine injury. This was different from the NLC because the NEXUS criteria do not consider the events surrounding the injury. Patients with blunt head or neck trauma were included in the study if they were alert [defined as a value of 15 on the Glasgow Coma Scale (GCS)] and stable (defined as systolic blood pressure

For Alert (Glasgow Coma Scale Score = 15) and Stable Trauma
Patients Where Cervical Spine (C-Spine) Injury is a Concern

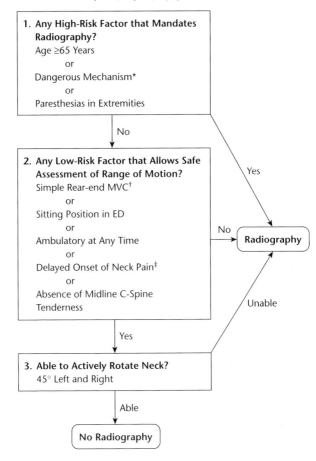

Figure 5.3 The Canadian C-spine rules. ED, emergency department; MVC, motor vehicle collision. (Source: *Journal of the American Medical Association* 2001; **286**:1841. Copyright © 2001, American Medical Association. All rights reserved.)

greater than 90 mmHg and respiratory rate greater than 10 but less than 24/min). Patients were excluded if they met one of the following predefined criteria: age less than 16 years; minor injuries, not including blunt head/neck trauma (such as lacerations or abrasions); GCS below 15; grossly abnormal vital signs; injury age of greater than 48 h; penetrating trauma; acute paralysis; known vertebral disease; return for reassessment of the same injury; or pregnancy.

Data were collected based on 20 standardized clinical findings from the neurologic status, patient history and physical examination. Patients underwent imaging of the cervical spine at the discretion of the treating physician. This was not mandatory and therefore some patients did not undergo imaging. For those patients without cervical spine imaging, a structured telephone follow-up was conducted to assess for missed injuries. The purpose of this hybridized gold standard was to ensure that there were no missed injuries in patients who did not receive radiographs. Patients were considered not to have a clinically significant cervical spine injury if, during the telephone interview at 14 days, they met all of the following criteria: (i) neck pain was rated as mild or none; (ii) restriction of neck movement was rated as mild or none; (iii) the use of a cervical collar was not required: and (iv) the neck injury did not prevent the return of the patient to their usual occupational activities.

The CCR includes three sets of criteria that need to be evaluated in a stepwise manner (Fig. 5.3). The stepwise nature of the CCR makes it somewhat more complicated than the NEXUS criteria and a bit more difficult to remember. However, if a patient satisfies all of the criteria, the decision rule indicates a low risk of cervical spine injury and radiography can be deferred. The following lists the criteria that must be fulfilled in order to safely defer imaging according to the CCR.

Criterion 1: Is there any high-risk factor that mandates radiography? Specifically, does the patient satisfy any of the following: age 65 years or older, paresthesias in any extremity, or a dangerous mechanism of injury (defined as a fall from 1 m or greater, axial load to the head as in a diving injury, motor vehicle crash at a speed in excess of 100 km/h, rollover or ejection, motorized recreational vehicle, bicycle collision)? If yes to any of these, radiographic imaging is recommended. If no, the second set of criteria are assessed.

Criterion 2: Are there any low-risk factors that allow safe assessment of a range of motion of the cervical spine? Specifically, are any of the following present: simple rear-end motor vehicle crash (excludes pushed into oncoming traffic, hit by bus/large truck, rollovers, hit by high-speed vehicle), sitting position in the ED, ambulatory at any time, delayed onset of neck pain (defined as not immediate onset of neck pain), or absence of midline cervical spine tenderness? If none of these are present, radiographic imaging is recommended. If any one of these is present, the final criterion is assessed.

Table 5.2 Canadian C-spine rule (CCR): study results and test performance from Stiell *et al.*[2]

Assessment result for any cervical injury	Radiographically documented injury		Decision rule performance	
	Injury	No injury		95% CI
Decision rule positive	151	5041	Sensitivity 100%	98–100
			Specificity 42.5%	40–44
Decision rule negative	0	3732	NPV 100%	99.9–100
			PPV 2.9%	2.5–3.4

NPV, negative predictive value; PPV, positive predictive value.

Criterion 3: Is the patient able to actively rotate their neck 45 degrees to the left and right? If no, radiographic imaging is recommended. If yes, the patient meets all of the criteria to safely forgo imaging of the cervical spine.

For the derivation study, a total of 12 782 patients were eligible; of those, 3281 patients were not enrolled and another 577 patients were excluded because they did not undergo imaging and could not be reached for follow-up. A total of 8924 patients were included in the final study group and had either radiographic imaging or the proxy 14-day telephone follow-up. The incidence of documented cervical spine injury in the study was low at 1.7%. Table 5.2 shows the study results and test performance.

Finally, Stiell and colleagues compared both sets of rules in a large prospective study in the same EDs that participated in the derivation study for the CCR.[3] The study aimed to compare the performances of the two rules (CCR vs. NLC) to determine which was the more specific and to validate the CCR. The methodologies for applying the clinical decision rules were the same as outlined in the original studies, but the inclusion and exclusion criteria of the CCR derivation study were used and not all patients underwent imaging (consistent with the CCR study but in contrast to the NLC study). The criteria for both sets of rules were prospectively determined and recorded prior to cervical spine imaging.

The authors achieved their objective of validating the CCR. Among the 8283 patients enrolled, 7438 had complete data from both sets of rules and underwent either cervical spine imaging or the 14-day telephone proxy instrument. The incidence of cervical spine injury in this study was 2%. Table 5.3 shows the test results and the test characteristics. In comparing the performance of the two rules, the authors found the CCR to have a higher sensitivity, negative predictive value (NPV), and specificity. Table 5.4 shows the results and performance of the NLC.

Table 5.3 Validation results of the Canadian C-spine rule (CCR) and test performance from Stiell et al.[3]

Assessment result	Radiographically documented injury		Decision rule performance	
	Injury	No injury		95% CI
Decision rule positive	161	3995	Sensitivity 99.4%	96–100
			Specificity 45%	44–46
Decision rule negative	1	3281	NPV 100%	99.8–100
			PPV 3.9%	3.3–4.5

NPV, negative predictive value; PPV, positive predictive value.

Table 5.4 NEXUS low-risk criteria (NLC): results and test performance from Stiell et al.[3]

Assessment result	Radiographically documented injury		Decision rule performance	
	Injury	No injury		95% CI
Decision rule positive	147	4599	Sensitivity 90.7%	85–94
			Specificity 36.8%	36–38
Decision rule negative	15	2677	NPV 99.4%	99–100
			PPV 3.1%	2.6–3.6

NPV, negative predictive value; PPV, positive predictive value.

Clinical question two

"How do the test performances of plain radiographs and CT of the cervical spine compare for identifying cervical spine injuries after blunt trauma?"
New high speed CT technology has resulted in more liberal use of this modality for cervical spine imaging. A meta-analysis from 2005 examined the English language literature from 1995 to 2004 and found seven studies in which both investigations were performed.[4] Studies had to have C-spine plain imaging with at least three standard views (anteroposterior, lateral, open mouth odontoid) and CT scanning that extended from occiput to the first thoracic vertebrae with a distance between images of less than 5 mm. The analysis examined 3834 patients and the prevalence of cervical spine injury was 11.7%. This prevalence is notably higher than in a general population of ED patients. Pooled sensitivity of plain radiography for detecting cervical spine injury was 52% (95% CI 47–56). The pooled sensitivity of CT scanning

of the cervical spine was 98% (95% CI 96–99). Specificity, positive and negative predictive values could not be calculated because there was no independent gold standard test. Injuries identified by CT were considered true injuries.

Comment

The NLC and the CCR have both been validated in large cohorts of patients in ED patients with blunt trauma to the neck. In the validation cohorts, both have high sensitivities (>99.3%) and negative predictive values (>99.9%), making both decision rules safe.

When comparing the two rules, Stiell and colleagues concluded that the CCR performed better than the NLC.[3] We feel that there are sufficient differences between the two rules and the studies supporting them to make the issue not as clear cut as Stiell has suggested. Table 5.5 compares and contrasts the differences in the derivation, validation, and implementation of these rules.

Given the differences, we believe that both sets of rule are useful for assessing the stable patient with blunt trauma. Overall, the NLC are somewhat easier to use clinically because they are less difficult to remember. The CCR are more complex and must be employed in a stepwise fashion. In our experience, the most common reason for failure of the NLC and for the need for cervical radiography is midline tenderness. The CCR are more specific than the NLC and patients with midline tenderness can be identified who do not otherwise meet criteria for cervical radiography.

Because of the higher specificity of the CCR, we propose that the CCR criteria be applied as a first step in the ED. While both the NLC and the CCR have roughly equal high sensitivity and high negative predictive values, CCR will have many fewer false positives. That is not to say that the NLC should not be used, just that you should be aware that while the NPV is very high with both sets of rules, the very low specificity of the NLC will lead to more unnecessary imaging (i.e. false positives—when the prediction rule indicates that the patient is not low risk and therefore recommends imaging).

We do however want to remind you that should there be a suspicion for cervical spine injury for any reason beyond those elements incorporated into either set of rules, you should err on the side of clinical safety and obtain imaging. A missed C-spine fracture can have catastrophic consequences to patients, including potential disability and even death. In the case of a negative rule but a high clinical suspicion of injury, clinical judgment should always be used when choosing whether to employ or defer cervical radiography.

Regarding whether or not plain films or CT should be the initial test of choice in blunt cervical trauma, it appears in the limited studies of highly

Table 5.5 A comparison of NEXUS low-risk criteria (NLC) and the Canadian C-spine rule (CCR)

	NLC	CCR	Comment
Explicit description for each criterion in the rule	Intoxication and painful distracting injury left undefined	High risk mechanism defined by the authors	NLC: • authors felt intoxication and painful distracting injury were best determined clinically and strict definitions would limit use in clinical practice CCR: • intoxication not included as it was found in the preliminary studies to not be predictive of injury • provided list of high-risk mechanisms but many others exist that are not explicitly listed
Patient enrollment	Patients with blunt trauma undergoing cervical imaging	Patients with complete data (undergoing either imaging or 14-day proxy telephone survey)	NLC: • risk of selection bias based on whether or not at risk patients got initial imaging, possibly limiting generalizability CCR: • not all patients had gold standard (imaging) but proxy tool accounted for those patient without imaging
Exclusion criteria	Patients with penetrating trauma or who had cervical imaging for reasons other than blunt trauma	List of excluded condition explicitly listed	Exclusion criteria limit generalizability NLC: • These are reasonable given the emphasis on blunt trauma CCR: • No explanation as to why age, pregnancy, and spinal disease were listed

Age criteria	None	Age 16 years or older	NLC: • no age limitation CCR: • excluded patients younger than 16 years, limiting generalizability
Incidence of clinically significant injury	2.4%	1.7%	
Study size (validation study)	>34 000 patients in 21 US medical centers	>7400 patients in nine Canadian medical centers	Diverse ED patient populations makes results generalizable
Sensitivity, % (validation study)	99% (95% CI 98–99.6)	99.4% (95% CI 96–100)	Comparable sensitivities, with correspondingly high NPVs
Specificity, % (validation study)	12.9% (95% CI 12.8–13)	45.1% (95% CI 44–46)	The CCR has a significantly higher specificity, therefore fewer false positives
Decision rule usability	Five elements to determine as present or absent	A total of three sets of criteria, totaling 14 elements to determine; some dictate imaging, others dictate no imaging	NLC: • fewer elements and a straightforward interpretation, is simpler to use CCR: • many elements makes it cumbersome to use • age criteria simplifies approach for older patients

NPV, negative predictive value.

selected trauma patients, CT C-spine has a higher sensitivity for detecting cervical spine injury compared to plain film imaging. However, in these studies, the overall prevalence of cervical spine injury was much higher than is seen in everyday ED practice. In fact, it was nearly six times higher than in the NEXUS and Canadian studies. This selection bias makes it difficult to generalize the patients in these studies (patients were enrolled at primary trauma centers) to the typical patient with a minor motor vehicle crash who is seen in the ED and outside of the trauma bay. Regardless, at this time, in patients suspected of C-spine injury, our opinion is that you should consider CT imaging over plain radiographs, especially in high-risk cases. However, radiation exposure and cost are the two factors that have not been sufficiently explored. While there may be subgroups of patients who would benefit from CT scanning over plain radiography, the data on this topic remains unclear.

References

1. Hoffman, J.R., Mower, W.R., Wolfson, A.B., Todd, K.H. and Zucker, M.I. (2000) Validity of a set of clinical criteria to rule out injury to the cervical spine in patients with blunt trauma. National Emergency Radiography Utilization Study Group. *New England Journal of Medicine* **343**(2): 94–99.
2. Stiell, I.G., Wells, G.A., Vandemheen, K.L., *et al.* (2001) The Canadian C-spine rule for radiography in alert and stable trauma patients. *Journal of the American Medical Association* **286**(15): 1841–1848.
3. Stiell, I.G., Clement, C.M., McKnight, R.D., *et al.* (2003) The Canadian C-spine rule versus the NEXUS low-risk criteria in patients with trauma. *New England Journal of Medicine* **349**(26): 2510–2518.
4. Holmes, J.F. and Akkinepalli, R. (2005) Computed tomography versus plain radiography to screen for cervical spine injury: a meta-analysis. *Journal of Trauma* **58**(5): 902–905.

Chapter 6 **Cervical Spine Fractures in Older Adults**

Highlights

- The prevalence of traumatic cervical spine injury in older adults is approximately double compared with younger patients.
- Clinical decision rules for determining who should undergo imaging of the cervical spine have excellent sensitivity but poor specificity.
- Clinicians should have a low threshold for imaging the cervical spine in older adults due to anatomic and physiologic changes that are less tolerant of even minor trauma.

Background

Older adults (≥65 years of age) presenting to the emergency department (ED) for evaluation after blunt trauma involving the neck should be evaluated for potential cervical spine injuries. Anatomic and physiologic factors associated with the older adult patient, such as osteopenia, osteophytes, and relative immobility, predispose them to cervical injury in the setting of low impact or minimal energy transfer mechanisms. In addition, one of the current clinical decision rules to identify patients who are at low-risk for clinically significant cervical spine injury—the Canadian C-spine rule (CCR)—identifies patients who are 65 years and older as a high-risk group who should receive objective radiography.

Clinical question

"Are there decision rules for determining low risk for cervical spine injury in older adults?"

Evidence-Based Emergency Care: Diagnostic Testing and Clinical Decision Rules. By J.M. Pines and W.W. Everett. Published 2008 by Blackwell Publishing, ISBN: 978-14051-5400-0.

Table 6.1 Performance of NEXUS low-risk criteria (NLC) among patients 80 years and older from Ngo et al.[1]

NEXUS	Radiographically documented injury			Decision rule performance	
	Injury	No injury	Total		95% CI
Decision rule positive	50	888	938	Sensitivity 100%	93–100
				Specificity 13%	11–15
Decision rule negative	0	132	132	NPV 100%	97–100
				PPV 5%	5–6
Total	50	1020	1070		

NPV, negative predictive value; PPV, positive predictive value.

There are three studies which address the issue of a clinical decision rule to identify older adults with a low risk of cervical spine injury. Two examine a subset of patients from the National Emergency X-Radiography Utilization Study (NEXUS): one group comprised patients that were considered very elderly ($\geq$80 years)[1] and the other included patients selected using a usual definition of elderly ($\geq$65 years).[2] A third study examined patients aged 65 years and older to stratify cervical spine injury risk in an effort to guide appropriate imaging.[3]

The first study was a subgroup analysis of 1070 patients from the NEXUS study that were 80 years or older.[1] The pre-defined study objective was to test the NEXUS low-risk criteria (NLC) performance in this very elderly population to determine the efficacy of the decision rule for obtaining cervical spine radiographs. The injury patterns were also examined. The prevalence of cervical spine injury in this older patient group was 4.7%, which was twice that of the total NEXUS cohort. Table 6.1 shows the test performance in this group.

No injuries were missed in this cohort. A total of 13% were correctly identified as being low risk, representing those who could possibly forgo cervical imaging. Injuries of the first and second cervical vertebra accounted for nearly half of all injuries (47%), in contrast to studies of younger patients in which the lower cervical spine is injured more frequently.

The second study was a subgroup analysis of 2943 patients from the NEXUS study that were 65 years or older.[2] The prevalence of cervical spine injury in this subgroup was 4.6%. The authors examined the performance of the NLC among this group and found that it had an overall sensitivity of 98.5% for any cervical injury and 100% for clinically significant cervical injury (Table 6.2).

Table 6.2 Performance of NEXUS low-risk criteria (NLC) among patients 65 years and older from Touger et al.[2]

	Sensitivity, % (95% CI)	Specificity, % (95% CI)	PPV (95% CI)	NPV (95% CI)
Assessment result for any cervical injury	98.5 (94.8–99.7)	14.6 (14.6–14.8)	5.3 (5.2–5.3)	99.5 (98.3–99.9)
Clinically significant cervical injury	100 (97.1–100)	14.7 (14.6–14.7)	4.9 (4.9–5.0)	100 (99.1–100)

NPV, negative predictive value; PPV, positive predictive value.

Cervical spine injuries occurred in a total of 135 geriatric patients, with the NLC identifying all but two injuries. Neither of the two injuries misclassified by the NLC required neurosurgical intervention. Analysis of the specific types of injuries occurring in the older population revealed that fractures of C1 and C2 represented more than half of all cervical fractures. Among the individual NEXUS criteria responsible for a patient to be classified as not low risk, midline tenderness (53%) and distracting injury (44%) were the most frequent.

Bub and colleagues performed a case-control study among trauma registry patients in Seattle from 1995–2002[3] specifically examining cervical spine fractures in elderly patients. The objective was to derive and validate a clinical decision rule identifying cervical spine fracture using clinical and history elements to guide imaging in high-risk patients aged 65 year and above.

Cases were identified from an inpatient trauma registry. Selection from all available cervical spine cases was not explicitly described, but only patients 65 years or older with non-penetrating trauma and who had confirmatory cervical imaging prior to death were eligible. Patients transferred to the trauma center were also excluded to minimize referral center bias. Controls were chosen from among ED patients seen between 1995 and 2002 (admitted or discharged) who were age 65 years or older, had blunt trauma with the absence of cervical fracture, and who were not transferred to the ED. Statistical methods included simple logistic regression, forward stepwise multivariable logistic regression modeling, recursive partitioning, receiver operator characteristic (ROC) curve analysis, and bootstrap validation techniques.

The incidence of cervical spine fracture was 2.6% among all the trauma registry patients examined during the study period (n = 3958). One hundred three cases and 107 control patient records were identified and included in the study. The final clinical prediction rule (Fig. 6.1) was able to stratify patients according to cervical fracture risk and used the author definitions (Table 6.3).

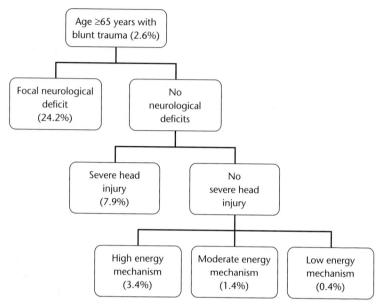

Figure 6.1 Schematic of clinical prediction rule for cervical spine fractures in elderly patients in a trauma registry from Bub *et al.*[3] Percentages correspond to absolute cervical fracture risk.

Table 6.3 Definitions for clinical prediction rule from Bub *et al.*[3]

Criterion	Definition
Severe head injury	• intracranial hemorrhage • skull fracture • unconscious • all intubated patients
High energy mechanism	• fall from a height of 10 feet • pedestrian struck by an automobile • airplane accident • high speed motor vehicle injury ($\geq$30 mph)
Moderate energy mechanism	• low speed motor vehicle injury (<30 mph) • fall from <10 feet • skiing accident
Low energy mechanism	• fall from standing or sitting position

Comment one

It is clinically intuitive that older patients can have spine injuries from mechanisms and situations that may be not obvious. Older patients can incur significant injuries from seemingly minor mechanisms such as falling out of a chair or falling from standing. Furthermore, older patients may not report symptoms or circumstances in as clear a manner as younger patients because of underlying medical illness, dementia, and/or difficulty in communicating. The two secondary analyses from the NEXUS group focus on cervical spine injuries in the elderly (≥65 years) and the very elderly (≥80 years). These two studies reveal that using the NLC patients at low risk of cervical spine injury can be identified with a very high sensitivity. While age is not an independent risk factor in the NEXUS criteria, you should use common sense and intuition as to the likelihood of a cervical spine injury in older adults. There has been one published case involving a 101-year-old patient in which applying the NEXUS criteria resulted in misclassifying a patient as being low risk for cervical spine injury.[4] The CCR, on the other hand, has an age criterion (≥65 years) that prompts imaging regardless of other risk factors. There has not been an independent study examining only elderly patients with blunt trauma or a subset analysis of elderly patients from the CCR study performed to date.

The clinical prediction rule developed by Bub *et al.*[3] has only been derived and validated in the same dataset. At this point, we would exercise caution in using this rule until it has been validated in an external setting. Additional limitations about clinical usefulness include the absence of both reported test performance characteristics and the need for cervical imaging, and only cervical spine fractures were identified. Furthermore, the rule itself is not explicitly intuitive in what it accomplishes, other than to stratify the risk of cervical fracture. The simple fact that all older patients are at risk of cervical fractures given the data extracted in their study implies a more liberal imaging tendency rather that a selective approach, which was the goal of both the NEXUS and CCR studies.

Comment two

Geriatric patients with blunt trauma may be assessed with the NLC in order to detect cervical spine injury with a high sensitivity. However, keep in mind the physiologic and anatomic changes that occur with aging together with the knowledge that less overall force is needed to incur a significant injury. When evaluating older adults with potential cervical spine trauma, we would recommend employing a very conservative approach because of the higher likelihood of clinically significant injuries, even in the context of minor trauma.

References

1. Ngo, B., Hoffman, J.R. and Mower, W.R. (2000) Cervical spine injury in the very elderly. *Emergency Radiology* 7(5): 287–291.
2. Touger, M., Gennis, P., Nathanson, N., *et al.* (2002) Validity of a decision rule to reduce cervical spine radiography in elderly patients with blunt trauma. *Annals of Emergency Medicine* **40**(3): 287–293.
3. Bub, L.D., Blackmore, C.C., Mann, F.A. and Lomoschitz, F.M. (2005) Cervical spine fracture in patients 65 years and older: a clinical prediction rule for blunt trauma. *Radiology* **234**(1): 143–149.
4. Barry, T.B. and McNamara, R.M. (2005) Clinical decision rules and cervical spine injury in an elderly patient: a word of caution. *Journal of Emergency Medicine* **29**(4): 433–436.

Chapter 7 **Cervical Spine Fractures in Children**

> **Highlights**
>
> - The prevalence of traumatic cervical spine injuries in children is less than 1%.
> - The National Emergency X-Radiography Utilization Study (NEXUS) low-risk criteria (NLC) are highly sensitive but poorly specific in children older than 8 years old.
> - There should be a low threshold for imaging nonverbal children and patients with suspicious or high energy injury mechanisms.
> - Large prospective studies are unlikely to be performed because of the low prevalence of cervical spine injuries in children.

Background

Cervical spine injury in the pediatric population is a major concern in the setting of blunt trauma, albeit less common relative to adults. Imaging of the cervical spine is frequently used in children; however, very few (<1%) of cases are positive for cervical spine injuries.

Clinical question

"Are there decision rules for determining low risk for cervical spine injury in the pediatric patient?"

There has been one large multicenter, prospective study carried out to examine a clinical decision rule for obtaining cervical spine radiographs in pediatric patients with blunt trauma.[1] The study comprised a pre-specified analysis of patients less than 18 years of age who were enrolled in NEXUS and involved applying the five-item NLC to them.[2] If none of the criteria were

Evidence-Based Emergency Care: Diagnostic Testing and Clinical Decision Rules. By J.M. Pines and W.W. Everett. Published 2008 by Blackwell Publishing, ISBN: 978-14051-5400-0.

Table 7.1 Test characteristics for the NEXUS low-risk criteria (NLC) in children from Viccellio et al.[1]

Assessment result for any cervical injury	Radiographically documented injury			Decision rule performance	
	Injury	No injury	Total		95% CI
Decision rule positive	30	2432	2462	Sensitivity 100%	87.8–100
Decision rule negative	0	603	603	Specificity 19.9%	18.5–21.3
				NPV 100%	99.2–100
Total	30	3035	3065	PPV 1.2%	0.8–1.8

NPV, negative predictive value; PPV, positive predictive value.

present, the patient was considered low risk for cervical spine injury. When any one of the criteria was positive, the patient was classified as not low risk, and the decision rule hence recommended cervical imaging. Only patients who underwent cervical imaging were included in NEXUS.

The NEXUS cohort was comprised of 34 069 patients and included 3065 pediatric patients (9% of the total study cohort). The incidence of cervical spine injury in the pediatric subgroup was 0.98% (n = 30). The distribution of injuries was mainly in the lower cervical spine.

Table 7.1 shows the performance of the NLC in children. A perfect sensitivity was achieved, but due the low number of actual injuries the confidence intervals were wide (95% CI: 88–100). The authors point out that of the 603 (approximately 20%) patients that the NLC classified as low risk (i.e. for whom the decision rule was negative), no cervical spine injury occurred.

Comment

In the only prospective study examining a decision rule regarding risk determination for cervical spine injury in children with blunt trauma, Viccellio et al. validated the NLC as being highly sensitive. Exploration of their data also found no cases of spinal cord injury without radiographic abnormality (SCIWORA) in any child, which is always a lingering concern in the minds of clinicians. The authors are careful to note that there were 3000 patients with 30 cervical spine injuries resulting in wide confidence intervals around the test parameters, despite not missing any case of cervical spine injury. They further report that it would require a study of nearly 80 000 children to narrow the confidence intervals to within 0.5%, making it highly unlikely they will ever improve on the current performance of the NLC in children.

A major concern clinicians may have is in applying the NLC in the infant (0–2 years) and toddler (2–8 years) groups, as they may be nonverbal or it may be difficult to accurately determine whether any individual item is present or absent. In fact, only 4 of the 30 cervical spine injuries occurred in patients ≤8 years old. Despite this concern, at least one criterion was positive among these four patients. Differences between the cervical spine anatomies are greatest during the infant/toddler and adolescent/adult developmental stages; this partially explains why more cervical spine injuries occur in the lower cervical spine in the younger age groups and in the higher cervical spine in the older age groups.

Because of the very low prevalence of cervical spine injury in patients of 8 years or younger and the impracticality of performing a larger study examining pediatric patients, clinicians should use clinical judgment in this younger age group. We recommend applying the NLC in the verbal and cooperative patients above 8 years old. You should take care to exercise vigilance in ruling out cervical spine injuries in children because missed injuries can lead to poor outcomes. If there is either a high-risk mechanism of injury or a high suspicion for cervical spine injury based on clinical evaluation, we certainly recommend obtaining objective neck imaging.

References

1. Viccellio, P., Simon, H., Pressman, B.D., *et al.* (2001) A prospective multicenter study of cervical spine injury in children. *Pediatrics* **108**(2): E20.
2. Hoffman, J.R., Mower, W.R., Wolfson, A.B., Todd, K.H. and Zucker, M.I. (2000) Validity of a set of clinical criteria to rule out injury to the cervical spine in patients with blunt trauma. National Emergency Radiography Utilization Study Group. *New England Journal of Medicine* **343**(2): 94–99.

Chapter 8 **Blunt Abdominal Trauma**

Highlights

- There are many diagnostic tests available to evaluate the presence of intra-abdominal injury in patients with blunt abdominal trauma including computed tomography (CT) scans, focused assessment by sonography in trauma (FAST), and diagnostic peritoneal lavage.
- FAST has high sensitivity and accuracy in adult patients and is a useful, rapid, non-invasive adjunct that is used routinely in the evaluation of blunt abdominal trauma.
- FAST is particularly useful in unstable trauma patients who cannot go immediately for CT imaging.
- High clinical suspicion in the setting of a negative FAST should prompt further evaluation by CT scanning or surgical exploration.
- Caution should be used with a negative FAST examination in pediatric trauma patients due to poor sensitivity in this population.

Background

In the acutely injured patient with abdominal trauma, many diagnostic modalities are available in the emergency department (ED) to detect the presence of solid organ injuries and intra-abdominal bleeding. There have been many studies comparing abdominal ultrasound (US) with CT scans, most of which have shown that CT is superior to US in detecting intra-abdominal injuries. CT scanning does have drawbacks, primarily in that it can not be safely performed in unstable patients. In order to detect the presence of intra-abdominal bleeding, a diagnostic peritoneal lavage can be used for patients that are too unstable for a CT scan. However, over the past ten years diagnostic

Evidence-Based Emergency Care: Diagnostic Testing and Clinical Decision Rules. By J.M. Pines and W.W. Everett. Published 2008 by Blackwell Publishing, ISBN: 978-14051-5400-0.

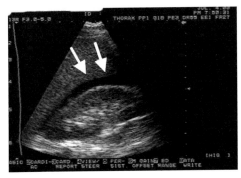

Figure 8.1 Patient involved in blunt trauma. The focused assessment by sonography in trauma (FAST) reveals fluid in Morison's Pouch (arrows). (Courtesy of Anthony Dean, MD.)

US in the form of a FAST examination has emerged as a safe, rapid, and non-invasive alternative to diagnostic peritoneal lavage in unstable patients in hospitals where an ED US is available (Fig. 8.1). While the FAST examination does not completely rule out the presence of intra-abdominal injuries—that is, it is not 100% sensitive—it is often used during the initial evaluation of trauma patients to provide early information regarding the presence of intra-abdominal bleeding.

Clinical question one

"How accurate is FAST compared to a CT scan in adult patients with blunt abdominal trauma?"
An early study that compared diagnostic peritoneal lavage to US and CT scans was performed in China.[1] Liu *et al.* compared the accuracy of the three modalities to detect significant intra-abdominal injuries in a prospective study. Patients with stable vital signs after their initial resuscitation and with equivocal physical examination findings underwent CT and US, followed by diagnostic peritoneal lavage. If any of the three examinations was positive the investigators performed a laparotomy. They used the surgical findings as the gold standard and compared this to the results of the diagnostic tests. For the 55 patients studied, the sensitivity, specificity, and accuracy of each of the tests are shown in Table 8.1.

The authors reported that a considerable issue in the use of US was the potential to miss small intestinal perforations. Since then, many studies have been performed evaluating the use of US in adults with blunt abdominal trauma (Table 8.2).

Table 8.1 Comparison of test sensitivity, specificity and accuracy of computed tomography (CT) scans, diagnostic peritoneal lavage (DPL), and ultrasound (US) in 55 patients, using surgical findings as the gold standard from Liu et al.[1]

	Sensitivity (%)	Specificity (%)	Accuracy (%)
CT scan	97.2	94.7	96.4
DPL	100.0	84.2	94.5
US	91.7	94.7	92.7

Table 8.2 Test performance summaries of ultrasound to detect intra-abdominal injury in blunt abdominal trauma

Authors	N	Patients	Sensitivity (%)	Specificity (%)	Accuracy (%)
Hoffmann et al.[2]	291	Severely injured (ISS >20)	89	97	94
McKenney et al.[3]	1000	Blunt trauma	88	99	97
Rothlin et al.[4]	312	Blunt thoracic and abdominal injury	90.1*	99.5	—
Rozyski et al.[5]	476	Blunt abdominal trauma	79	95.6	—
Dolich et al.[6]	2576	Blunt abdominal trauma	86	98	97

* 98.1% for intra-abdominal fluid and 41.4% for solid organ injuries. ISS, injury severity score.

A systematic review performed in 2001 aimed to determine the precision and reliability of US in blunt abdominal trauma.[7] The authors performed a statistical analysis and reported summary receiver operating characteristic curves (SROCs) using weighted and robust regression models, with Q* denoting the shoulder of the curve, and calculated post-test probabilities as a function of pooled likelihood ratios (LRs). They found that 30 of 123 trials were eligible for their enrollment; these included data on 9047 patients. They also found that ultrasonography showed a summary Q* value of 0.91 (where 1.0 represents perfect sensitivity and specificity) and negative predictive values ranged from 72 to 99%. For screening for free fluid, the SROC was calculated at Q* = 0.89. They found that US detects the presence of organ lesions, but does not adequately exclude abdominal injuries (LR− = 0.23). They calculated that given a pre-test probability of 50% (0.5) for blunt abdominal injury, a post-test probability of nearly 25% (0.25) remains in the case of a negative US. They concluded that despite high specificity, US has a low sensitivity for the detection of both free fluid and solid organ lesions. In cases where there is a suspicion of true intra-abdominal injury (i.e. a high pre-test probability), they concluded that another assessment (e.g. CT scan) must be performed regardless of the initial US findings.

Clinical question two

"Can FAST exclude intra-abdominal injuries in pediatric patients with blunt trauma?"
Three studies have examined the sensitivity of FAST in detecting intra-abdominal injuries in pediatric patients requiring laparotomy.[8–10] In these studies, sensitivities ranged from 33 to 55%. Another study by Luks *et al.* reported a higher US sensitivity of 89% in a pediatric population; however, a gold standard examination was not performed in all patients.[11]

Comment

The FAST examination performs with high sensitivity in the detection of hemoperitoneum and is therefore useful in blunt abdominal trauma patients who are unstable. In many Level I trauma centers, FAST has become a useful adjunct in nearly all patients with blunt abdominal trauma—not just the unstable patients, and is part of the evaluation process following the primary and secondary surveys. In centers where US is readily available, it has all but replaced diagnostic peritoneal lavage in unstable trauma patients with potential hemoperitoneum. In cases of a high pre-test probability when there is a suspicion of solid organ injury, and in children, the FAST examination should not be used as a gold standard and further testing or laparotomy should be considered in consultation with a trauma surgeon.

References

1. Liu, M., Lee, C.H. and P'eng, F.K. (1993) Prospective comparison of diagnostic peritoneal lavage, computed tomographic scanning, and ultrasonography for the diagnosis of blunt abdominal trauma. *Journal of Trauma* **35**: 267–270.
2. Hoffmann, R., Nerlich, M., Muggia-Sullam, M., *et al.* (1992) Blunt abdominal trauma in cases of multiple trauma evaluated by ultrasonography: a prospective analysis of 291 patients. *Journal of Trauma* **32**: 452–458.
3. McKenney, M.G., Martin, L., Lentz, K., *et al.* (1996) 1000 consecutive ultrasounds for blunt abdominal trauma. *Journal of Trauma* **40**: 607–610; discussion 611–612.
4. Rothlin, M.A, Naf, R., Amgwerd, M., *et al.* (1993) Ultrasound in blunt abdominal and thoracic trauma. *Journal of Trauma* **34**(4): 488–495.

5. Rozycki, G.S., Ochsner, M.G., Jaffin, J.H., *et al.* (1993) Prospective evaluation of surgeons' use of ultrasound in the evaluation of trauma patients. *Journal of Trauma* **34**: 516–26; discussion 526–527.

6. Dolich, M.O., McKenney, M.G., Varela, J.E., *et al.* (2001) 2576 ultrasounds for blunt abdominal trauma. *Journal of Trauma* **50**(1): 108–112.

7. Stengel, D., Bauwens, K., Sehouli, J., *et al.* (2001) Systematic review and meta-analysis of emergency ultrasonography for blunt abdominal trauma. *British Journal of Surgery* **88**(7): 901–912.

8. Patel, J.C. and Tepas, J.J. (1999) The efficacy of focused abdominal sonography for trauma (FAST) as a screening tool in the assessment of injured children. *Journal of Pediatric Surgery* **34**: 44–47; discussion 52–54.

9. Mutabagani, K.H., Coley, B.D., Zumberge, N., *et al.* (1999) Preliminary experience with focused abdominal sonography for trauma (FAST) in children: is it useful? *Journal of Pediatric Surgery* **34**: 48–52; discussion 52–54.

10. Coley, B.D., Mutabagani, K.H., Martin, L.C., *et al.* (2000) Focused abdominal sonography for trauma (FAST) in children with blunt abdominal trauma. *Journal of Trauma* **48**: 902–906.

11. Luks, F.I., Lemire, A., St-Vil, D., *et al.* (1993) Blunt abdominal trauma in children: the practical value of ultrasonography. *Journal of Trauma* **34**: 607–611.

Chapter 9 **Acute Knee Injuries**

> **Highlights**
>
> - Acute knee fractures are identified in a small proportion of emergency department (ED) patients with acute knee injuries.
> - The Ottawa knee rule (OKR) and Pittsburg knee rule (PKR) are highly sensitive in guiding the need for imaging in adults and children with acute knee injuries

Background

Acute knee injuries are a common complaint in emergency medicine practice. Before the advent of clinical decision rules, the usual practice was to order plain radiographs of the knee to rule out a fracture in the patients with blunt trauma and a clinical suspicion of fracture. Similar to ankle injuries, knee fractures are only identified in a small proportion of cases (about 7%). Two clinical decision rules have been created to identify patients in which knee radiography may be deferred in patients with blunt knee trauma: the Ottawa knee rule (OKR) and the Pittsburgh knee rule (PKR).

The OKR recommend knee radiography if any of the following are present in the context of an acute knee injury:
- age 55 years or older;
- tenderness at the head of fibula;
- isolated tenderness at the patella;
- inability to flex knee to 90 degrees; or
- inability to transfer weight for four steps both immediately after the injury and in the ED.

Evidence-Based Emergency Care: Diagnostic Testing and Clinical Decision Rules. By J.M. Pines and W.W. Everett. Published 2008 by Blackwell Publishing, ISBN: 978-14051-5400-0.

Exclusion criteria for the OKR include: age <18, superficial skin injuries, injuries greater than seven days old, re-evaluation of recent injuries, altered levels of consciousness, paraplegia, or multiple injuries.

The PKR recommends radiography if the mechanism of injury is either blunt trauma or a fall and either:

1. Age less than 12 years or above 50 years; or
2. there is an inability to walk four weight-bearing steps in the ED.

Exclusion criteria for the PKR are knee injuries occurring more than six days before presentation, only superficial lacerations and abrasions, a history of previous surgeries or fractures on the injured knee, and those being reassessed for the same injury.

Clinical question one

"How well do the OKR work in identifying patients that require knee radiography?"

This question was addressed in a recent systematic review of studies on the OKR, which included articles that reported patient information to determine levels of sensitivity and specificity.[1] Two independent reviewers independently tallied data on study samples, the ways that the OKR was used, and methodological characteristics. There were 11 studies identified; the data from six, involving 4249 adult patients, were considered appropriate for pooled analysis. The results of this analysis were that the negative likelihood ratio was 0.05 (95% CI: 0.02–0.23), sensitivity was 98.5% (95% CI: 93.2–100), and specificity was 48.6% (95% CI: 43.4–51.0). Given a knee fracture prevalence of 7%, if the OKR are negative, this gives a probability of knee fracture of 1.5%. Table 9.1 shows the data from the six studies reviewed, with reported sensitivities and specificities.

Table 9.1 Six studies reporting sensitivity and specificity of the Ottawa knee rules

Reference	Year	Sensitivity, % (95% CI)	Specificity, % (95% CI)
Steill[2]	1996	100 (94–100)	50 (46–53)
Steill[3]	1997	100 (94–100)	48 (45–51)
Richman[4]	1997	85 (65–96)	45 (39–52)
Emparanza[5]	2001	100 (96–100)	52 (50–55)
Szucs[6]	2001	100 (63–100)	47 (36–58)
Ketelslegers[7]	2002	100 (87–100)	32 (26–38)

Clinical question two

"How do the OKR compare with the PKR?"

A prospective study conducted at three academic centers investigated this question.[8] The decision whether to order radiographs was made based on the judgment of the physician. All patients that underwent radiography had a four-view knee series (one anterior-posterior, one lateral, and two oblique) and a sunrise view added when patellar fractures were suspected. The performance of the OKR and PKR was determined by using appropriate variables from the data sheets and film reports from board-certified radiologists. There were a total of 934 patients evaluated and the OKR and the PKR were applicable to 745 and 750 patients, respectively. The main results of the study are detailed in Table 9.2.

The difference in sensitivity was not significant; however, the PKR was considerably more specific (33% difference; 95% CI: 28–38). However, two elements of this study bring into question its validity. First, the authors failed to follow patients who did not undergo radiography, thus introducing a potential selection bias. However, in a previous study 357 patients with knee pain who did not have radiography were re-evaluated by a formal telephone interview two weeks later and none required clinical reassessment. A second issue was that two of the three clinical sites were University of Pittsburgh-affiliated hospitals. Therefore, it is possible that the individual physicians may have already been using the PKR or OKR to make decisions in following normal procedures for determining who needed knee films.

Table 9.2 Study comparing the Ottawa knee rules (OKR) with the Pittsburgh knee rules (PKR) from Seaberg *et al.*[8]

	NPV (%)	Sensitivity, % (95% CI)	Specificity, % (95% CI)	PPV (%)
PKR	99.8	99 (94–100)	60 (56–64)	24.1
OKR	98.5	97 (90–99)	27 (23–30)	14.8

NPV, negative predictive value; PPV, positive predictive value

Clinical question three

"How well do the OKR work in pediatric patients?"

A recent study aimed to determine the sensitivity and specificity of the OKR in children.[9] The authors performed a prospective, multicenter validation study and included children aged 2 to 16 years presenting to the ED with a knee injury sustained within the previous seven days. Physicians ordered radiographs according to their usual practice and the outcome measure was any fracture. Patients with negative films were followed for 14 days. A total of 750 were enrolled, 670 had radiography, and less than 10% (n = 70) had fractures. The OKR were 100% sensitive (95% CI: 95–100), with a specificity of 42.8% (95% CI: 39–47). The authors concluded that the OKR is valid to use in children.

Comment

When deciding whether or not to order a knee film in the ED, both the PKR and the OKR can be used to identify adults and children who may not need knee films in the setting of an acute knee injury. The PKR is considerably more specific and includes the mechanism of injury, which is an important feature for predicting fractures. Blunt knee injuries, including direct blows to the knee and falls, account for 80% of knee fractures. When this type of injury is present, patients are four-times more likely to have fractures.[10] While the specificity of the PKR is higher and may therefore result in less unnecessary radiography, the sensitivity for both rules was near 100%, making both safe for use in the ED. In addition, the OKR were determined safe for use in one study in children.

References

1. Bachmann, L.M., Haberzeth, S., Steurer, J., et al. (2004) The accuracy of the Ottawa knee rule to rule out knee fractures: a systematic review. *Annals of International Medicine* **140**: 121–124.
2. Stiell, I.G., Greenberg, G.H., Wells, G.A., et al. (1996) Prospective validation of a decision rule for the use of radiography in acute knee injuries. *Journal of the American Medical Association* **275**: 611–615.
3. Stiell, I.G., Wells, G.A., Hoag, R.H., et al. (1997) Implementation of the Ottawa knee rule for the use of radiography in acute knee injuries. *Journal of the American Medical Association* **278**: 2075–2079.
4. Richman, P.B., McCuskey, C.F., Nashed, A., et al. (1997) Performance of two clinical decision rules for knee radiography. *Journal of Emergency Medicine* **15**: 459–463.
5. Emparanza, J.I. and Aginaga, J.R. (2001) Validation of the Ottawa knee rules. *Annals of Emergency Medicine* **38**: 364–368.
6. Szucs, P.A., Richman, P.B. and Mandell, M. (2001) Triage nurse application of the Ottawa knee rule. *Academic Emergency Medicine* **8**: 112–116.
7. Ketelslegers, E., Collard, X., Vande Berg, B., et al. (2002) Validation of the Ottawa knee rules in an emergency teaching centre. *European Radiology* **12**: 1218–1220.

8. Seaberg, D.C., Yealy, D.M., Lukens, T., *et al.* (1998) Multicenter comparison of two clinical decision rules for the use of radiography in acute, high-risk knee injuries. *Annals of Emergency Medicine* **32**: 8–13.

9. Bulloch, B., Neto, G., Plint, A., *et al.* (2003) Validation of the Ottawa knee rule in children: a multicenter study. *Annals of Emergency Medicine* **42**: 48–55.

10. Dalinka, M.K., Alazraki, N.P., Daffner, R.H., *et al.* (2005) Expert Panel on Musculoskeletal Imaging. Suspected ankle fractures. *American College of Radiology* [WWW document]. URL http://www.guideline.gov/summary/summary.aspx?doc_id=8301

Chapter 10 **Blunt Head Injury**

Highlights

- The prevalence of computed tomography (CT) head scans that are positive for clinically significant injury in the emergency department (ED) population with minor head trauma is low.
- The New Orleans criteria (NOC) and Canadian CT head rule (CCHR) are sensitive clinical decision rules that identify patients at low risk for clinically significant head injuries where noncontrast head CT can be deferred.
- No decision rules have identified a population of older adults who are at low risk for intracranial injuries following head trauma.

Background

There are more than 1.5 million cases of traumatic head injuries occurring annually in the US, with a mortality rate of 3–4%. Patients with minor head injury, variably described as those having a Glasgow coma scale (GCS) score of 13–15 and a non-focal neurological examination, comprise the majority of traumatic head injury cases seen and evaluated in EDs. Traditionally, patients who have either a high-risk head injury or a loss of consciousness are evaluated with the use of noncontrast head CT to identify fractures, intracranial bleeding, and other clinically significant injuries (Fig. 10.1). However, the overall prevalence of clinically significant injuries is low in the ED population. Recent studies have focused on the identification of clinical factors that influence the likelihood of intracranial injury and researchers have constructed clinical decision rules to identify patients that do not require evaluation with noncontrast head CT.

Evidence-Based Emergency Care: Diagnostic Testing and Clinical Decision Rules. By J.M. Pines and W.W. Everett. Published 2008 by Blackwell Publishing, ISBN: 978-14051-5400-0.

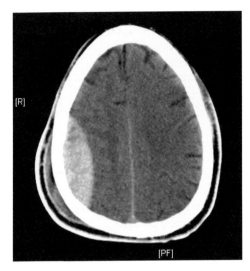

Figure 10.1 Epidural hematoma from a blunt head injury.

Clinical question one

"Which patients do not need a head CT after sustaining a minor head injury?"
Five well-designed and large prospective studies have evaluated this question.[1–5] The first of these to examine the problem and to create a set of clinical decision rules, known as the New Orleans criteria (NOC), was published in 2000 by Haydel *et al.*[1] In this study, patients presenting to a single inner-city ED were examined in order to identify those with minor head injury who did not need to undergo noncontrast head CT. Enrolled patients were three years old or above, had loss of consciousness or amnesia after the incident, had normal neurological examinations, and a GCS of 15. A total of 1429 patients were enrolled in the study and all underwent head CT. The initial portion of the study was a derivation phase that included 520 patients. Eight clinical findings collected during the study were determined *a priori* by the study authors as being associated with significant head injury. These included headache, age greater than 60 years, vomiting, drug or alcohol intoxication, deficits in short-term memory, post-traumatic seizure, coagulopathy, or evidence of trauma above the clavicles. Each criterion was explicitly defined by the authors. The presence or absence of each factor was determined before the head CT was performed. Head CTs were interpreted by radiologist who did not have information about the clinical criteria being assessed. A positive

head CT included acute intracranial hemorrhages and hematomas, cerebral contusions, and depressed skull fractures. An analysis of the eight clinical factors determined that the presence of any one of seven factors yielded a decision rule that was 100% sensitive. The final set of clinical criteria that were tested on a validation cohort (n = 909) were as follows:

- headache;
- age 60 years or older;
- vomiting;
- drug or alcohol intoxication;
- short-term memory loss;
- seizure after the injury; and
- evidence of trauma above the clavicles.

The test results and decision rule performance are shown in Table 10.1.

Within a year of publishing the NOC, Canadian researchers led by Ian Stiell introduced the Canadian CT head rule (CCHR).[2] This study examined patients presenting to 10 Canadian EDs within 24 hours of sustaining a blunt head trauma who had loss of consciousness, amnesia, or disorientation, and an initial GCS of 13 or above, in order to determine two outcome measures: the need for neurosurgical intervention (death and neurosurgical procedures)

Table 10.1 Performance of the New Orleans criteria (NOC) in the derivation and validation phases from Haydel *et al.*[1]

NOC derivation cohort (n = 520)	Head CT result			Decision rule performance	
	Injury	No injury	Total		95% CI
Decision rule positive (≥1 factor present)	36	368	404	Sensitivity 100%	90–100
				Specificity 24%	
Decision rule negative (all factors absent)	0	116	116	NPV 100%	20–28
				PPV 9%	
Total	36	484	520		
NOC validation cohort (n = 909)	Injury	No injury	Total		
Decision rule positive	57	640	697	Sensitivity 100%	96–100
				Specificity 25%	
Decision rule negative	0	212	212	NPV 100%	6–12
				PPV 8%	
Total	57	852	909		

CT, computed tomography; NPV, negative predictive value; PPV, positive predictive value.

and clinically important brain injury requiring hospital admission and neurological follow-up (abnormal head CT requiring admission). Patients underwent either head CT or a structured outpatient telephone evaluation. The study employed derivation methods to examine 22 clinical factors in each patient. The larger set of variables was ultimately distilled into a final set of seven clinical variables using statistical validation techniques. The seven risk factors were broken down into two categories according to the outcome. Five were used to classify patients as high risk for neurosurgical intervention:

- GCS score of less than 15 at 2 hours after injury;
- suspected open or depressed skull fracture;
- two or more episodes of vomiting after injury;
- any sign of basal skull fracture; and
- age 65 years or above.

Two more variables were added in order to classify patients as medium risk for brain injury on head CT:

- amnesia before impact of greater than 30 minutes; and
- dangerous mechanism (pedestrian struck by motor vehicle, ejection from motor vehicle, fall from a height of more than 3 ft or five stairs).

Only patients with complete data were included in the analysis. The study enrolled 3121 patients over three years. The overall prevalence of neurosurgical intervention and brain injury on CT was 1.4 and 8.1%, respectively. When all five high-risk factors were absent, no injuries requiring neurosurgical interventions were missed, yielding a negative predictive value (NPV) of 100% (95% CI: 99–100; Table 10.2). When all seven risk factors were absent, four intracranial injuries were missed, none requiring interventions, yielding a NPV of 99% (95% CI: 99.2–99.9; Table 10.2).

Canadian researchers followed the derivation/validation study with a head-to-head study comparing the NOC with the CCHR.[3] The study was performed in nine Canadian EDs and enrolled more than 2000 patients with over 300 practicing physicians involved. To make a fair, direct comparison of the two clinical decision rules only the patients with a GCS of 15 were included; however, an analysis of the CCHR on the larger cohort was also performed (i.e. including patients with GCS of 13 or 14). Prior to carrying out a head CT scan, physicians completed a data form that included both the NOC and CCHR. Outcomes were need for neurosurgical intervention and clinically important brain injuries, similar to the prior study. Patients not undergoing head CT were followed up with a 14-day telephone interview. Only patients with complete data receiving head CT, or with complete data and a 14-day follow-up if they did not receive a head CT, were included for analysis. The incidence of neurosurgical intervention and clinically important brain injury was 0.4 and 5.3%, respectively.

Table 10.2 Test performance of the Canadian computed tomography head rule (CCHR) from Stiell *et al.*[2]

CCHR high risk (five factors)	Need for neurosurgical intervention			Decision rule performance	
	Yes	No	Total		95% CI
Decision rule positive (≥1 factor present)	44	962	1006	Sensitivity 100%	92–100
				Specificity 69%	67–70
Decision rule negative (all factors absent)	0	2115	2115	NPV 100%	99–100
				PPV 4%	3–5
Total	44	3077	3121		

CCHR medium risk (all seven factors)	Any clinically important brain injury			Decision rule performance	
	Yes	No	Total		95% CI
Decision rule positive	250	1446	1696	Sensitivity 98%	96–99
				Specificity 50%	47–51
Decision rule negative	4	1421	1425	NPV 99%	99.2–99.9
				PPV 14%	13–16
Total	254	2867	3121		

NPV, negative predictive value; PPV, positive predictive value.

Table 10.3 illustrates the test performance for each clinical decision rule. Both rules performed with very high sensitivities (100%) and did not miss any injuries. Applying the NOC resulted in significantly more false positives (i.e. the rule indicated that the patient was not at low risk and the head CT showed no injury), which yielded a lower specificity. The authors concluded that given the equivalent sensitivities, using the CCHR would be likely to result in fewer head CTs being ordered.

An external validation study of the NOC and CCHR for head-injured patients was performed in a large Dutch study between 2002 and 2004 (see Table 10.4).[4] This multicenter trial included four university hospitals and a total of 3181 patients were enrolled with blunt head trauma. Patients had to present within 24 hours of sustaining the injury, have a GSC of 13 or above, and have at least one of the following risk factors: a reported loss of consciousness, amnesia, short-term memory loss, post-traumatic seizure, severe headache, vomiting, an appearance of being intoxicated with alcohol or drugs, physical evidence of injury above the clavicles, current warfarin use

Table 10.3 Comparison of clinical decision rules for patients with a GCS of 15 from Stiell et al.[3]

Need for neurosurgical intervention	CCHR			NOC		
	Injury	No injury	Total	Injury	No injury	Total
Decision rule positive	8	430	438	8	1595	1603
Decision rule negative	0	1384	1384	0	219	219
Total	8	1814	1822	8	1814	1822
Sensitivity (95% CI)	100% (63–100);			100% (63–100);		
Specificity (95% CI)	76.3% (74–78)			12% (10–13)		
NPV (95% CI)	100% (99–100);			100% (98–100);		
PPV (95% CI)	1.8% (0.8–4)			0.5% (0.2–1)		

Any clinically important brain injury	CCHR			NOC		
	Injury	No injury	Total	Injury	No injury	Total
Decision rule positive	97	853	950	97	1506	1603
Decision rule negative	0	872	872	0	219	219
Total	97	1725	1822	97	1725	1822
Sensitivity (95% CI)	100% (96–100);			100% (96–100);		
Specificity (95% CI)	50% (48–53)			12% (11–14)		
NPV (95% CI)	100% (99–100);			100% (98–100);		
PPV (95% CI)	10% (8–12)			6% (5–7)		

CCHR, Canadian computed tomography head rule; GCS, Glasgow coma scale; NOC, New Orleans criteria; NPV, negative predictive value; PPV, positive predictive value.

or a history of coagulopathy, or to have a neurological deficit. Note that all seven of the NOC criteria are included in the enrollment criteria for this study. Given the differences in the inclusion criteria based on GCS, a separate analysis was made for each clinical prediction rule based on the original description. All patients included in the study underwent head CT and the interpreting radiologist was not blinded to the data being collected. Physician assessment was performed by a neurologist prior to head CT. The outcomes were need for neurosurgical intervention within 30 days of the traumatic injury, and traumatic injury detected on CT requiring hospitalization.

The authors concluded that both the NOC and CCHR performed with 100% sensitivity, despite the application in a new setting and the slight differences in the strictly-defined inclusion/exclusion criteria, and also the explicit definitions for each criterion in each rule. The specificities were much lower for each rule and may not result in fewer head CTs being ordered.

Table 10.4 External validation results comparing two clinical decision rules performances on a Dutch patient cohort with head injuries from Smits et al.[4]

Need for neurosurgical intervention	CCHR			NOC		
	Injury	No injury	Total	Injury	No injury	Total
Decision rule positive	7	1269	1276	2	1236	1238
Decision rule negative	0	752	752	0	69	69
Total	7	2021	2028	2	1305	1307
Sensitivity (95% CI)	100% (59–100);			100% (15–100);		
Specificity (95% CI)	37% (35–39)			5% (4–6)		
NPV (95% CI)	100% (99–100);			100% (94–100);		
PPV (95% CI)	0.5% (0.2–1)			0.1% (0–0.6)		
Neurocranial traumatic CT finding	Injury	No injury	Total	Injury	No injury	Total
Decision rule positive	171	1105	1276	115	1152	1267
Decision rule negative	34	718	752	2	67	69
Total	205	1823	2028	117	1219	1336
Sensitivity (95% CI)	83% (77–88);			98% (94–99);		
Specificity (95% CI)	39% (37–41)			5% (4–7)		
NPV (95% CI)	95% (93–97);			97% (90–99);		
PPV (95% CI)	13% (11–15)			9% (7–11)		

CCHR, Canadian computed tomography head rule; CT, computed tomography; GCS, Glasgow coma scale; NOC, New Orleans criteria; NPV, negative predictive value; PPV, positive predictive value.

The largest study to date to derive a clinical decision rule to identify patients that are low risk for having intracranial injuries after blunt trauma came from the National Emergency X-Radiography Utilization Study (NEXUS) II group.[5] Patients were enrolled between 1999 and 2000 and the results were published in October 2005. The study consisted of a multicenter, prospective, observational study in 21 EDs of patients presenting with blunt trauma for which a head CT was ordered. Detailed clinical and mechanistic information on 19 variables was collected and recorded by physicians prior to head CT. Patients not undergoing head CT at the discretion of the treating physician were not included in the study. The two outcomes that were examined were the presence of a significant intracranial injury, defined as the need for neurosurgical intervention that might otherwise lead to a precipitous deterioration or long-term neurological impairment, and minor head injuries, defined as intracranial injuries among patients with a GCS of 15. This was a derivation study that used recursive partitioning to select the set of clinical predictors that would maximize the sensitivity while optimizing the specificity. No patient follow-up was described. A total of 13 728 patients were enrolled, including 917 patients with intracranial injuries, of whom 330 had a GCS of 15. Eight clinical variables were chosen that yielded the highest sensitivity with maximal specificity:

- evidence of significant skull fracture;
- scalp hematoma;
- neurological deficit;
- age 65 years and above;
- altered level of consciousness;
- abnormal behavior;
- coagulopathy; and
- persistent vomiting.

The performance of the NEXUS II head CT (HCT) rules is shown in Table 10.5. The highest sensitivity that was achieved for detecting any

Table 10.5 Performance of the NEXUS II head computed tomography (HCT) rule from the derivation study from Mower et al.[5]

	NEXUS II HCT rules all intracranial injuries		
	Injury	No injury	Total
Decision rule positive	901	11 059	11 960
Decision rule negative	16	1 752	1 768
Total	917	12 811	13 728
Sensitivity (95% CI)		98% (97–99)	
Specificity (95% CI)		13% (13–14)	
NPV (95% CI)		99% (98–99.5)	
PPV (95% CI)		7.5% (7–8)	

	NEXUS II HCT rules minor head injury (GCS 15)		
	Injury	No injury	Total
Decision rule positive	314	8 375	8 689
Decision rule negative	16	1 752	1 768
Total	330	10 127	10 457
Sensitivity (95% CI)		95% (92–97)	
Specificity (95% CI)		17% (16–18)	
NPV (95% CI)		99% (98–99.5)	
PPV (95% CI)		3.6% (3–4)	

GCS, Glasgow coma scale; NPV, negative predictive value; PPV, positive predictive value.

intracranial injury was 98% (95% CI: 97–99) with a specificity of 13% (95% CI: 13–14). The authors concluded that the eight clinical factors were good discriminators for identifying patients at high risk for traumatic brain injury. However, they also acknowledged that a prospective validation study was needed to further confirm their clinical prediction instrument.

Comments

Minor head injuries are a common ED complaint with a low prevalence of clinically significant injury and/or need for intervention following non-contrast head CT. Because the prevalence of injury is low, head CTs are often negative for these patients. The estimated prevalence of injury varies from 0.5 to 4% across the US. The CCHR and the NOC have been proposed to differentiate those who need a head CT after minor head injury from those who do not.

Since the introduction of these two clinical decision rules, both have been reproduced and externally validated. Stiell and colleagues compared the two rules in a head-to-head study and found the sensitivities for both to be 100%.[3] The specificities differed significantly, however, implying that fewer head CTs would be averted if applying only the NOC. The original NOC study was criticized as not having any patient follow-up after discharge from the ED. This element is at least partially addressed in this comparison study, which included outpatient follow-up for all of those patients not undergoing head CT. An inherent bias of the comparison study is the use of EDs that were included in the development and derivation/validation studies, hence leading to an enhanced familiarity with the CCHR over the NOC, despite the author's explanation to the contrary. But readers should find reassurance that overall, the two rules appropriately detected those patients with clinically meaningful traumatic cranial injuries.

The NEXUS II HCT rules have only been derived and not validated, therefore we cannot comment on their performance beyond the findings in the original study. Readers will take specific note, however, of the similarity between the three sets of decision rules. All include evidence of head trauma, elderly patients, and vomiting as high-risk factors. Therefore regardless of which rule is ultimately used, it is safe to assume that each of these factors is concerning and not unique to the study setting.

The application of a decision rule in a clinical setting significantly different from the one it was derived in is a major test in determining the ultimate usefulness of the rule in clinical practice. Dutch researchers took on the challenge and studied the performances of each clinical decision rule in Dutch patients with head injuries.[4] The difficulties of adapting a clinical decision rule to already established practice standards were handled well in this study. Each rule performed with 100% sensitivity for detecting the need for neurosurgical intervention. The NOC had higher sensitivities for CT-detected injuries than did the CCHR, which the authors felt was likely to be because of the restrictive definition for physical evidence of head trauma (only signs of basilar skull fracture or depressed skull fracture) in contrast to the broader criterion in the NOC (any evidence of trauma above the clavicles). In contrast, the specificities of the NOC were significantly lower than both the original study and the comparison by Stiell *et al.* This is because all of the NOC were included among the list of conditions a patient had to meet for eligibility.

Regardless, at this point the studies have shown the reproducibility and external validation of the rules in detecting the most important intracranial injuries. What remains to be seen are the results of a formal impact analysis that will determine if clinicians will actually use the rules and what their impact will be on ordering head CTs. Inconsistencies in the inclusion/exclusion criteria between studies, the absence of head CTs for all patients in the Canadian-based studies, and the ever-present legal ramifications of not wanting to miss any intracranial injuries, raise concerns of translation of these results into confident clinical practice application.

A conservative approach that we suggest is to apply both the NOC and the CCHR to an individual patient. While it is more difficult to remember two rules than one, the overall sensitivity is likely to be higher if both are applied. If one or more of the risk factors are present, a head CT would be recommended. Additionally, if clinical judgment or other factors not described in these studies are present and the patient might have a serious injury, a head CT is warranted. However, the absence of all risk factors suggests an extremely low chance of a clinically significant head injury. Care should be taken to use clinical judgment when deciding what is or is not a dangerous mechanism and in making a reasonable judgment about whether their injury justifies a head CT. Furthermore, we would recommend strict follow-up precautions in all patients with minor head injuries and blunt head traumas, particularly those for whom a head CT was not ordered.

Clinical question two

"Are there decision rules for determining low risk for intracranial injury in the elderly patient?"

There are no decision rules that have studied elderly patients in order to determine if they are at low risk of intracranial injury. There is an advanced age criterion in the NOC (>60 years old), the CCHR (≥65 years old), and the

NEXUS II HCT rules, designating these patients at high risk in the setting of blunt trauma. It is unlikely that future studies will focus exclusively on the elderly in this clinical context. Anatomic changes associated with aging include smaller brain volumes that predispose the patient to the development of hemorrhages. Changes in cognition as well as medication use (most notably antiplatelet agents, anticoagulants, and antihypertensive agents) place the elderly patient at potentially higher risk for traumatic injuries from mechanisms such as falls, in addition to the normal trauma mechanisms. Therefore, a clinical practice that includes obtaining a head CT for all patients with blunt head trauma who are elderly is supported by these authors.

References

1. Haydel, M.J., Preston, C.A., Mills, T.J., Luber, S., Bladeau, E. and DeBlieux, P.M.C. (2000) Indications for computed tomography in patients with minor head injury. *New England Journal of Medicine* **343**(2): 100–105.
2. Stiell, I.G., Wells, G.A., Vandemheen, K., *et al.* (2001) The Canadian CT head rule for patients with minor head injury. *Lancet* **357**: 1391–1396.
3. Stiell, I.G., Clement, C.M., Rowe, B.H., *et al.* (2005) Comparison of the Canadian CT head rule and the New Orleans criteria in patients with minor head injury. *Journal of the American Medical Association* **294**(12): 1511–1518.
4. Smits, M., Dippel, D.W.J., de Haan, G.G., *et al.* (2005) External validation of the Canadian CT head rule and the New Orleans criteria for CT scanning in patients with minor head injury. *Journal of the American Medical Association* **294**(12): 1519–1525.
5. Mower, W.R., Hoffman, J.R., Herbert, M., Wolfson, A.B., Pollack, C.V. and Zucker, M.I. (2005) Developing a decision instrument to guide computed tomographic imaging of blunt head injury patients. *Journal of Trauma* **59**(4): 954–959.

Chapter 11 **Blunt Head Trauma in Children**

Highlights

- Blunt head trauma in children is associated with significant morbidity and mortality.
- Four sets of clinical decision rules to identify children at high risk of intracranial injury from blunt head trauma have been derived: University of California-Davis head computed tomography (HCT) rules, National Emergency X-Radiography Utilization Study (NEXUS) II HCT rules, children's head injury algorithm for the prediction of important clinical events (CHALICE) rules, and the Italian pediatric HCT rules.
- All are highly sensitive but none have been prospectively validated.

Background

Traumatic brain injury is a leading cause of morbidity and mortality in children and accounts for a significant proportion of ED visits and hospitalizations annually, which total in excess of one million for all trauma-related head injuries. The concern of the physician seeing a child involved in a trauma is to establish the presence or absence of an intracranial injury. Efforts in North America and Europe have addressed the development of clinical decision rules for children with blunt head traumas to establish criteria to identify patients who would be considered not low risk, and therefore for whom head computed tomography (CT) imaging would be recommended.

Clinical question

"Are there decision rules for determining low risk for intracranial injury in pediatric patients?"

Evidence-Based Emergency Care: Diagnostic Testing and Clinical Decision Rules. By J.M. Pines and W.W. Everett. Published 2008 by Blackwell Publishing, ISBN: 978-14051-5400-0.

In examining the available studies, we reviewed only prospective studies. There are four large studies in children that have derived sets of clinical variables in order to identify those who are at low risk of intracranial injury.[1-4] The first study from researchers at the University of California-Davis enrolled patients younger than 18 years with a history of recent blunt head trauma. Children presenting with falls from ground level, running into stationary objects with abrasions only, or patients transferred from other facilities with head CT already completed, were excluded. After patients were evaluated by a physician, data forms were completed prior to the patient going to head CT. Imaging was left to the discretion of the treating physician and therefore not all patients underwent imaging. All admitted patients were followed throughout their hospital stay to determine if an outcome event occurred. Patients discharged from the ED were contacted by telephone one week later. Mailed questionnaires went out to those who were not reached by telephone. Finally, morgue and trauma registry records were reviewed to determine outcome events for those not reached by phone or survey. Two outcomes were assessed. The first was traumatic brain injury identified on CT, defined as intracranial hemorrhage, hematoma, or cerebral edema (isolated skull fracture was not considered by the authors because they do not require hospitalization). The second was traumatic brain injury requiring intervention, defined as needing any of the following: a neurosurgical procedure, anticonvulsant therapy for more than one week, or two nights or more of hospitalization for treatment of the head injury.

The study enrolled 2043 children over three years old (1999–2001). Head CT imaging was performed in 62% (n = 1271) of the patients. The prevalence of the two outcomes—traumatic brain injury on CT and traumatic brain injury requiring intervention—were 7.7% (98/1271) and 5.1% (105/2043), respectively. A complete follow-up via telephone interview or survey was obtained for 88% of patients. Through the use of recursive partitioning methods, a decision rule was derived for the detection of both outcomes. Five variables included in the decision rule included: abnormal mental status, clinical signs of skull fracture, a history of vomiting, headache, and scalp hematoma in children aged two years or younger. Four of the five variables were assessed with high inter-observer agreement ($k \geq 0.67$). Only scalp hematoma had a lower inter-observer agreement ($k = 0.53$), but this was included because it was highly predictive in the youngest patients. Table 11.1 shows the performance of the five factors in the decision rule on the two separate outcomes.

In a preplanned analysis of the National Emergency X-Radiography Utilization Study (NEXUS) II investigation, Oman *et al.* studied patients aged 18 years or younger to examine the performance of the NEXUS II low-risk

Table 11.1 Performance measures of the University of California (UC)-Davis head computed tomography (HCT) rules for the derivation cohort from Palchak et al.[1]

	UC-Davis HCT rules: traumatic brain injury on CT			Decision rule performance	
	Injury	No injury	Total		95% CI
Decision rule positive	97	870	967	Sensitivity 99%	94–100
				Specificity 26%	23–28
Decision rule negative	1	303	304	NPV 99.7%	99–100
				PPV 10%	8–12
Total	98	1173	1271		

	UC-Davis HCT rules: traumatic brain injury requiring intervention			Decision rule performance	
	Injury	No injury	Total		95% CI
Decision rule positive	105	1111	1216	Sensitivity 100%	97–100
				Specificity 43%	40–45
Decision rule negative	0	827	827	NPV 100%	99–100
				PPV 8.6%	7–10
Total	105	1938	2043		

NPV, negative predictive value; PPV, positive predictive value.

head CT (HCT) rules on this population.[2] The NEXUS II HCT rules are described in detail in Chapter 10 (see Table 10.5 for performance results). In an adaptation suited for the study of children, only seven of the eight variables were evaluated (the advanced age criterion was dropped). NEXUS II enrolled 1666 children, all of whom underwent head CT. The outcomes evaluated were the same as for the larger NEXUS II study; i.e. clinically important intracranial injury (ICI) that required neurosurgical intervention or was likely to lead to significant long-term neurological impairment. The prevalence of clinically significant ICI was 8.3% (138/1666). The performance of the adapted NEXUS II HCT rules is shown in Table 11.2. Readers must keep in mind that in this study the NEXUS II authors have used a decision rule that was derived using a large cohort of patients (n = 13 728), and are now presenting results of how that clinical decision rule performs in a subset of the original study group. Therefore, it is not surprising that sensitivities are very high and the specificity is low, similar to the original NEXUS II study results.

Table 11.2 Performance of the National Emergency X-Radiography Utilization Study (NEXUS) II head computed tomography (HCT) rule in children from Oman et al.[2]

	NEXUS II HCT rules: clinically important ICI			Decision rule performance	
	Injury	No injury	Total		95% CI
Decision rule positive	136	1298	1434	Sensitivity 98%	95–100
				Specificity 15%	13–17
Decision rule negative	2	230	232	NPV 99%	97–100
				PPV 9%	97–100
Total	138	1528	1666		

	NEXUS II HCT rules: clinically important ICI – age <3 years			Decision rule performance	
	Injury	No injury	Total		95% CI
Decision rule positive	25	269	294	Sensitivity 100%	86–100
				Specificity 5%	3–9
Decision rule negative	0	15	15	NPV 100%	78–100
				PPV 8%	5–12
Total	25	284	309		

ICI, intracranial injury; NPV, negative predictive value; PPV, positive predictive value.

British researchers, also searching for a set of clinical predictors to identify children at low risk for clinically significant injury, created the children's head injury algorithm for the prediction of important clinical events (CHALICE) rule.[3] This study examined children under 16 years old between 2000 and 2002 that presented to EDs in 10 hospitals in the northwest of England with any history or sign of head injury. Only patients who refused to consent were excluded. Data was collected based upon 40 clinical variables. The primary outcome was a composite of death from head injury, requirement for neurosurgical intervention, or marked abnormality on head CT. Abnormalities in CT imaging were defined as an acute, new traumatic ICI that included intracranial hematomas, cerebral contusions, cerebral edema, and depressed skull fractures. Non-depressed skull fractures were specifically not included as they were deemed not significant injuries and do not normally require intervention or hospitalization. Similar to the Canadian CT head rule, the study did not mandate that all patients underwent CT. Patients who were admitted for inpatient stays, had a head CT or skull radiographs, or who underwent neurosurgery were followed up. At the end of the study all participating hospital radiology records were reviewed for skull radiographs and head CTs, and were cross-referenced with enrolled patients. The National Office of Statistics was also contacted regarding deaths in children with head injury. Recursive partitioning techniques were used to derive a set of clinical variables that would yield the highest possible sensitivity while trying to achieve maximal specificity.

This study, which is the largest of its kind dedicated to examining children, enrolled 22 772 patients. Only 744 patients underwent head CT. The prevalence of clinically significant head injury was 1.2% (281/22 772). The CHALICE rule states that a head CT is indicated if the patient has:

- a witnessed loss of consciousness lasting more than 5 min;
- a history of amnesia with a duration in excess of 5 min;
- abnormal drowsiness;
- three of more episodes of vomiting after the injury;
- a suspicion of non-accidental injury; or
- a seizure after injury.

Or if following examination any of the following are reported:

- a GCS of less than 14, or less than15 if younger than 12 months old;
- a suspicion of penetrating or depressed skull fracture, or bulging fontanelle;
- signs of basal skull fracture;
- focal neurological findings; or
- a bruise, swelling, or laceration in excess of 5 cm if younger than 12 months old.

Or if the mechanism for injury is any of the following:

- a high speed road traffic injury (>40 mph);
- a fall from a height in excess of 3 m (10 ft); or
- a high speed injury from a projectile or object.

It consists of 14 criteria, with a head CT being indicated when any item is present. In this derivation study, the clinical prediction rule for detecting any clinically significant head injury performed with a sensitivity of 98.6% and a specificity of 86.9% (Table 11.3).

A group from Italy examined a cohort of children under 16 years old involved in blunt head trauma presenting to pediatric EDs to determine predictors of the diagnosis of ICI and death.[4] They enrolled 3806 patients between 1996 and 1997 and derived a clinical prediction rule with five clinical variables. All patients discharged from the ED were followed up by phone after 10 days. Patients underwent routine care and ordering a head CT was at the discretion of the treating physician. The final variables included in the prediction model include loss of consciousness, drowsiness, amnesia, prolonged headache, and evidence of basal or non-frontal skull fracture. The presence of any one of these clinical variables would classify a patient as high

Table 11.3 Test performance of the children's head injury algorithm for the prediction of important clinical events (CHALICE) rule from Dunning *et al.*[3]

	Clinically significant head injury			Decision rule performance	
	Injury	No injury	Total		95% CI
CHALICE rule positive	277	2 933	3 210	Sensitivity 98.6%	96.4–99.6
				Specificity 86.9%	86.5–87.4
CHALICE rule negative	4	19 558	19 562	NPV 99.9%	99.9–100
				PPV 8.6%	7.7–9.7
Total	281	22 491	22 772		

NPV, negative predictive value; PPV, positive predictive value.

risk for death or intracranial injury. The absence of these variables classifies a patient as low risk for the outcomes. The performance of the derived model is shown in Table 11.4.

Comments

There are a growing number of high quality studies regarding pediatric patients with blunt trauma that seek to identify children at low risk for clinically significant head injuries. The four studies that have generated clinical prediction rules for identifying patients with intracranial injuries have, as yet, only been derived and none have been prospectively validated. Yet from the four large prospective cohort studies common themes regarding

Table 11.4 Test performance of the derivation phase of the Italian pediatric head computed tomography (HCT) rules from Da Dalt *et al.*[4]

	Clinically significant intracranial injury or death			Decision rule performance	
	Positive	Negative	Total		95% CI
Clinical decision rule positive	22	478	500	Sensitivity 100%	84–100
				Specificity 87%	86–88
Clinical decision rule negative	0	3298	3298	NPV 100%	99–100
				PPV 4%	2–7
Total	22	3776	3798[a]		

[a] Eight children with negative outcomes had no initial evaluation and therefore are not included. NPV, negative predictive value; PPV, positive predictive value.

the clinical variables that appear to be predictive emerge (Table 11.5). The only distinct unique variable found across all four rules was a clinical sign of skull fracture. Vomiting is included in three of the rules, along with scalp hematomas and abnormalities in mental status or behavior. Headache and specific mechanism of injury are both only included in one rule. The specific

Table 11.5 Summary of clinical variables included in the available pediatric head injury decision rules

UC-Davis[1]	NEXUS II[2]	CHALICE[3]	Italian pediatric ICI rule[4]
Abnormal mental status	Evidence of significant skull fracture	Witnessed LOC >5 min	Loss of consciousness
Clinical signs of skull fracture	Scalp hematoma	History of amnesia >5 min duration	Drowsiness
History of vomiting	Neurological deficit	Abnormal drowsiness	Amnesia
Headache	Altered level of consciousness	≥ three episodes of vomiting after injury	Prolonged headache
Scalp hematoma in child ≤2 years old	Abnormal behavior	Suspicion of non-accidental injury	Basal or non-frontal skull fracture
	Coagulopathy	Seizure after injury	
	Persistent vomiting	GCS <14 or GCS <15 if <12 months old	
		Suspicion of penetrating or depressed skull fracture, or bulging fontanelle	
		Signs of basal skull fracture	
		Focal neurological finding	
		Bruise, swelling, or laceration >5 cm if <12 months old	
		High speed road traffic injury (>40 mph)	

CHALICE, children's head injury algorithm for the prediction of important clinical events; GCC, Glascow coma scale; ICI, intracranial injury; LOC, loss of consciousness; NEXUS, National Emergency X-Radiography Utilization Study; UC-Davis, University of California-Davis wording of each clinical variable differs between the rules and can influence the performance and utility of the specific rule.[5] While these studies involved separate pediatric populations in different countries across a span of years, it is likely that these are the important clinical variables that clinicians should elicit until validation and implementation studies are available. The prevalence of intracranial injury in the studies ranged from 0.6–8.3%, and differs partially based on the definition of an injury. There is already evidence in the US that ordering patterns of head CTs for pediatric patients with blunt head trauma is increasing, and therefore the impact of evidence-based guidelines could be significant.

Not every child evaluated will require a head CT. Associated with every CT that is ordered are concerns over radiation exposure, the need for sedation in the youngest patients, and time away or out of the ED. Issues of cost are important, but are secondary to the clinical issues of concern in our perspective and should not be part of the decision-making process. Until validation and impact studies become available we recommend attention to the clinical factors listed in Table 11.5.

References

1. Palchak, M.J., Holmes, J.F., Vance, C.W., *et al.* (2003) A decision rule for identifying children at low risk for brain injury after blunt head trauma. *Annals of Emergency Medicine* **42**(4): 492–506.
2. Oman, J.A., Cooper, R.J., Holmes, J.F., *et al.*, and for the NEXUS II Investigators. (2006) Performance of a decision rule to predict need for computed tomography among children with blunt head trauma. *Pediatrics* **117**(2): 238–246.
3. Dunning, J., Daly, J.P., Lomas, J.P., Lecky, F., Batchelor, J., Mackway-Jones, K., and on behalf of the children's head injury algorithm for the prediction of important clinical events (CHALICE) study group. (2006) Derivation of the children's head injury algorithm for the prediction of important clinical events decision rule for head injury in children. *Archives of Disease in Childhood* **91**: 885–891.
4. Da Dalt, L., Marchi, A.G., Laudizi, L., *et al.* (2006) Predictors of intracranial injuries in children after blunt head trauma. *European Journal of Pediatrics* **165**: 142–148.
5. Sun, B.C., Hoffman, J.R. and Mower, W.R. (2007) Evaluation of a modified prediction instrument to identify significant pediatric intracranial injury after blunt head trauma. *Annals of Emergency Medicine* **49**: 325–32.

Chapter 12 **Acute Ankle and Foot Injuries**

Highlights

- The prevalence of ankle fractures among emergency department (ED) patients with ankle sprain is about 15%.
- The Ottawa ankle rules (OAR) are a widely used, well-validated set of clinical decision rules that accurately identify patients at low risk for fractures.
- The OAR have been shown to be highly sensitive in children; however, they should be used in populations that can give a good verbal history of the injury and that were able to walk prior to the injury.

Background

The management of patients with acute foot and ankle injuries is a common part of emergency medicine practice. The most common presentation is an inversion injury. Patients with these sorts of injuries can either have ankle fractures, which are typically seen on a three-view ankle series, or foot fractures, which are seen on a three-view foot series. Depending on the site of the injury and degree of tenderness, patients traditionally get an ankle series, a foot series, or both. However, the overall prevalence of fractures is relatively low (about 15% of injuries). The recognition that a high proportion of X-rays are negative in patients with these injuries triggered the development of the Ottawa ankle rules (OAR). The OAR were derived for the sensitivity to be 100%, so that if the criteria for the rules are met, fractures can be effectively ruled out based on the clinical evaluation and hence radiography can be deferred.

Evidence-Based Emergency Care: Diagnostic Testing and Clinical Decision Rules. By J.M. Pines and W.W. Everett. Published 2008 by Blackwell Publishing, ISBN: 978-14051-5400-0.

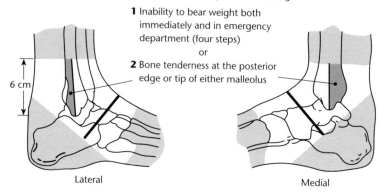

An ankle X-ray series is only necessary if there is pain near the malleoli and any of these findings:

1 Inability to bear weight both immediately and in emergency department (four steps)

or

2 Bone tenderness at the posterior edge or tip of either malleolus

6 cm

Lateral

Medial

Figure 12.1 The Ottawa ankle rules. (Source: *Journal of the American Medical Association* 1993; **269**:1127. Copyright © 1993, American Medical Association. All rights reserved.)

For ankle radiography to be deferred the patient must undergo physical examination of ankle and must meet two criteria (Fig. 12.1):
- ability to bear weight (four steps) immediately after the injury or in the ED; and
- absence of localized tenderness over the posterior aspect of either the distal lateral or distal medial malleolus.

For foot radiography to be deferred, the patient must undergo a physical examination and must meet two criteria (Fig. 12.2):
- ability to bear weight (four steps) immediately after the injury or in the ED; and
- absence of localized tenderness over the navicular or the base of the fifth metatarsal.

In the OAR studies, patients were excluded if they had a delayed presentation of injury (greater than one week), altered mental status, or were pregnant.

The OAR is probably the best studied of all decision rules in emergency medicine. The rules have been derived and validated in multiple settings across multiple cultures. The purpose of this chapter will be to briefly review the evidence behind the OAR and to examine the use of the OAR in children.

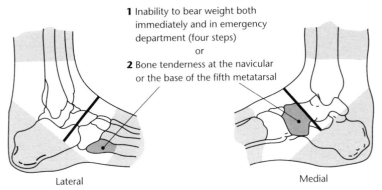

A foot X-ray series is only necessary if there is pain in the mid-foot and any of these findings:

1 Inability to bear weight both immediately and in emergency department (four steps)

or

2 Bone tenderness at the navicular or the base of the fifth metatarsal

Lateral   Medial

Figure 12.2 The Ottawa foot rules. (Source: *Journal of the American Medical Association* 1993; **269**:1127. Copyright © 1993, American Medical Association. All rights reserved.)

Clinical question one

"What is the extent of the evidence behind using the OAR to clinically exclude fractures of the ankle and mid-foot?"

In 2003, Bachmann *et al.* performed a systematic review and meta-analysis of the evidence behind the use of the OAR.[1] The authors extracted data on the study population, the type of OAR used, and study methodology. The intent was to calculate a pooled sensitivity for the decision rules. A bootstrapping method for statistical analysis was to ensure that their estimate of the standard error was correct. They also calculated and pooled negative likelihood ratios for many subgroups and adjusted for methodological quality. They excluded studies that had unknown blinding of the radiologist and those that were not prospective. For the 32 studies that met the inclusion criteria and 27 reporting data on 15 581 patients, they calculated a negative likelihood ratio of 0.08 (95% CI: 0.03–0.18) for the ankle and 0.08 (95% CI: 0.03–0.20) for the mid-foot. In children, the pooled negative likelihood ratio was 0.07 (95% CI: 0.03–0.18). The data in Table 12.1 were tabulated as bootstrapped sensitivities and specificities with a focus on specific populations, prevalence of fracture, and time to referral ('n' denotes the number of studies used to calculate the point estimate for the sensitivity or the median specificity.)

The authors calculated that applying these ratios to a 15% fracture prevalence yielded a less than 1.4% probability of actual fracture in these subgroups. The authors concluded that evidence supports the use of the OAR

Table 12.1 Sensitivities and specificities of the OAR in pooled studies from Bachmann *et al.*[1]

Category	Sensitivity, % (95% CI)	Median specificity, % (interquartile range)
All studies (n = 39)	97.6 (96.4–98.9)	31.5 (23.8–44.4)
Type of assessment:		
ankle (n = 15)	98.0 (96.3–99.3)	39.8 (27.9–47.7)
foot (n = 10)	99.0 (97.3–100)	37.8 (24.7–70.1)
combined (n = 14)	96.4 (93.8–98.6)	26.3 (19.4–34.3)
Population:		
children (n = 7)	99.3 (98.3–100)	26.7 (23.8–35.6)
adults (n = 32)	97.3 (95.7–98.6)	36.6 (22.3–46.1)
Prevalence of fracture:		
<25th centile (n = 7)	99.0 (98.3–100)	47.9 (42.3–77.1)
25–75th centile (n = 22)	97.7 (95.9–99.0)	30.1 (23.8–40.1)
>75th centile (n = 10)	96.7 (94.2–99.2)	27.3 (15.5–40.0)
Time to referral (hours):		
<48 (n = 5)	99.6 (98.2–100)	27.9 (24.7–31.5)
>48 (n = 34)	97.3 (95.9–98.5)	36.6 (19.9–46.8)

as an accurate tool to exclude fractures of the mid-foot and ankle with a close to 100% sensitivity and low specificity.

Clinical question two

"Can the OAR be used safely in children to exclude ankle and foot fractures?"
Safe application of the OAR in children has been the subject of recent debate. Three major considerations in children differentiate the use of the OAR in children from the safe practice in adults. The first issue is that children may not be as reliable regarding the verbal history of the injury. The most common missed fracture is a Salter-Harris type I fracture, which is defined as a separation of the bone 0.3 mm through the physis. Because Salter-Harris type I fractures are often associated with trauma in infants and children, point tenderness will generally be present if the patient is able to communicate. The third issue is that children must be able to walk prior to injury, in order for the OAR to be applied. This will exclude infants and children who are unable to ambulate.

In support of the high estimate for the sensitivity of the OAR in the seven pediatric studies in the systematic review by Bachmann *et al.*, a more recent review including additional data has reported good sensitivity of the OAR in children.[2] In the latter study, the authors calculated an overall sensitivity of 97% (95% CI: 93–100) and specificity of 29% (95% CI: 18–40). In all of the studies examined a prevalence of 12% was calculated. While one article in their review showed that a total of five patients who were rule negative actually had a fracture, yielding a sensitivity of 83% (95% CI: 65–94),[3] most articles had zero or one missed fracture in the pediatric population.

Comment

The OAR are very useful for clinically excluding fractures in both adult and pediatric populations and they have been validated in multiple settings. In applying the OAR to children, is important to only use the rules when children are able to communicate verbally and have the ability to walk prior to the injury. In the pooled studies reviewed in this chapter, a small percentage of the patients that were excluded from receiving X-rays based on the OAR did actually have a fracture. However, given a prevalence of 12% in pediatric studies and 15% in adult studies, a very low percentage of patients (less than 1.4%) will fall into this category. It is also unknown what the clinical relevance is of a subtle missed ankle fracture. Therefore, in the case of either negative ankle radiography or deferred ankle radiography because the patient did not meet the OAR, we recommend that patients with significant soft tissue injuries be splinted, use ice and elevation, and use crutches to minimize the discomfort of weight-bearing.

In the pediatric population, missed fractures will be of the Salter-Harris type I classification, which has almost no long-term consequence. As a note of caution, because the sensitivity for the rule is not 100%, in settings where the rule is negative and the pre-test probability is high, clinicians should use their best judgment in the decision to order foot and ankle X-rays.

References

1. Bachmann, L.M., Kolb, E., Koller, M.T., *et al.* (2003) Accuracy of Ottawa ankle rules to exclude fractures of the ankle and mid-foot: systematic review. *British Medical Journal* **326**(7386): 417.

2. Myers, A., Kanty, K. and Nelson, T. (2005) Are the Ottawa ankle rules helpful in ruling out the need for X-ray examination in children? *Archives of Disease in Childhood* **90**: 1309–1311.

3. Clarke, K.D. and Tanner, S. (2003) Evaluation of Ottawa ankle rules in children. *Pediatrics in Emergency Care* **19**: 73–78.

Chapter 13 **Occult Scaphoid Fractures**

Highlights

- Suspicion of scaphoid fracture is based on the mechanism of injury (fall on outstretched hand) and physical examination findings.
- Plain radiography will miss 5–20% of initial scaphoid fractures in the emergency department (ED).
- Missed scaphoid fractures can be associated with poor outcomes, including non-union, delayed union, and avascular necrosis.
- Patients with negative films should be splinted using a thumb spica.
- Close follow-up should be planned for patients with potential scaphoid fractures for follow-up re-evaluation, which may involve a repeat examination or radiographic testing.
- MRI seems to be the most sensitive test for occult scaphoid fractures.

Background

The scaphoid, also commonly known as the carpal navicular, is the most frequently fractured carpal bone, accounting for approximately 70–80% of all carpal fractures. Suspicion of a scaphoid fracture is based largely on a patient's mechanism of injury, which in most cases is from a fall on an outstretched hand (FOOSH). While not occurring exclusively in adolescence and early adulthood, scaphoid fractures have their highest incidence in these age groups. Scaphoid fractures occur infrequently in the very old and very young. Physical findings, such as tenderness in the anatomic snuffbox, pain with axial loading of the ipsilateral thumb, and pain with supination against resistance, have all been used as indications of a scaphoid fracture. Clinicians

---

Evidence-Based Emergency Care: Diagnostic Testing and Clinical Decision Rules. By J.M. Pines and W.W. Everett. Published 2008 by Blackwell Publishing, ISBN: 978-14051-5400-0.

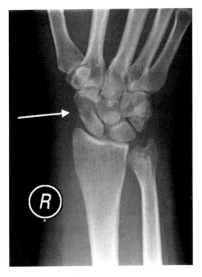

Figure 13.1 Scaphoid fracture (arrow).

should maintain a high level of suspicion when either a compatible mechanism is described (i.e. a FOOSH injury) or if any of the associated signs are present. The scaphoid bone has a retrograde blood supply, and therefore failure to diagnose a scaphoid fracture in the ED can result in avascular necrosis, non-union and delayed union, all of which can result in varying degrees of degenerative osteoarthritis and arthrosis. As a result, plain radiography is extensively used as the initial diagnostic modality and detects upwards of 80–95% of all scaphoid injuries (Fig. 13.1).

Four- and six-view plain X-ray series of the scaphoid have been proposed as the appropriate initial detection measures. In 5–20% of patients with a suspected fracture despite negative initial X-rays, follow-up plain X-rays within 5–14 days reveal the fracture in approximately 10–15% of cases. But for those patients still suspected of having a scaphoid fracture after negative films in the ED, referral for follow-up imaging is appropriate. Computed tomography (CT), bone scintigraphy (BS), and magnetic resonance imaging (MRI) are the typical options that might be considered for follow-up imaging. For patients with documented scaphoid fractures, referral to a hand surgeon and prompt treatment of the wrist injury in the ED is recommended. Such treatment includes immobilizing the suspected injury with a thumb spica splint or other similar splint while determining the next appropriate method of investigation.

Clinical question

"Which diagnostic imaging modality is recommended next for a clinically suspected scaphoid fracture when the initial plain X-rays are negative or non-diagnostic?"

Comparative studies for scaphoid fractures have focused on BS versus MRI. CT is generally not used when either BS or MRI is available, and therefore will not be discussed here. Similarly, studies examining the potential of ultrasound in diagnosing scaphoid fractures are starting to appear; however, these studies are limited based on sample sizes and diagnostic availability, and are also not recommended at this time.

Studies of the optimal diagnostic modality to use for a suspected occult scaphoid fracture with negative initial X-rays have compared MRI and BS. The largest of the studies involved 61 patients with wrist injuries that had negative initial and 7–10 day follow-up X-rays. BS and MRI each detected four additional scaphoid fractures.[1] Table 13.1 shows the diagnostic test characteristics for MRI and BS using a composite gold standard of MRI, BS, and follow-up X-rays.

Kitis *et al.* compared MRI and BS results performed 2–4 weeks after the initial assessment in 22 patients with suspected scaphoid injuries but with negative plain films.[2] Scaphoid fractures were identified in three patients by both MRI and BS; bone scanning detected one scaphoid fracture that MRI missed. Ten other non-scaphoid injuries were detected by MRI but not by BS. The authors concluded that both were sensitive tests, but that MRI had greater specificity for non-scaphoid injuries.

A small study in the Netherlands examined 16 patients with suspected occult scaphoid fractures using both MRI and BS, with the latter being

Table 13.1 Comparative studies of magnetic resonance imaging (MRI) and bone scintigraphy (BS) in the detection of occult scaphoid fractures

Reference Study	n	TP	TN	FP	FN	Sensitivity (95% CI)	Specificity (95% CI)
MRI*	43	6	37	0	0	100% (54–100)	100% (94–100)
BS*	43	5	35	2	1	83% (35–100)	95% (82–99)
MRI^	16	6	6	4	0	60% (26–87)	100% (54–100)

FN, false negative; FP, false positive; TN, true negative; TP, true positive.

* From Fowler *et al.* 1998. The gold standard is considered to be a composite of either BS-positive (for MRI comparison) or MRI-positive (for BS comparison) and all X-rays.

^ From Tiel-van Buul *et al.* 1996. The gold standard is considered to be BS.

considered the gold standard.[3] MRI had a sensitivity of 60% and a specificity of 100% (see Table 13.1), indicating that this technique was not superior to BS. While the sensitivity was calculated as 60%, only one true false negative occurred with MRI testing. Other MRI negative but BS positive patients were considered based on the nonspecific BS readings. It is clear from this study that MRI was able to delineate soft tissue and ligamentous injuries that were not clear on BS.

Finally, Thorpe *et al.* studied 59 patients in the UK with suspected occult scaphoid fractures using both MRI and BS.[4] All four scaphoid fractures identified by BS were also identified on MRI, plus other fractures. Three significant ligamentous injuries were diagnosed through MRI but were not seen on BS.

Comments

While plain X-rays detect the majority of scaphoid fractures on the initial evaluation, the long-term disability and the complications that arise from non-union or avascular necrosis are worrisome for clinicians. Repeat plain films in 7–10 days should detect a few fractures. The initial management remains similar for definite and suspected but not proven scaphoid injuries, but debate over the next appropriate diagnostic study to order varies.

Based on the series of small studies examining both MRI and BS, it appears that MRI is as sensitive as BS and has superior specificity for detecting occult scaphoid fractures. MRI has the additional benefit of discretely differentiating a soft tissue and ligamentous injury from a true bony injury with remarkable detail compared with bone scanning. Furthermore, the MRI results can be used to help guide surgical intervention if indicated. Therefore MRI should be the preferred follow-up diagnostic imaging study. MRI availability in the ED is typically not an issue in this case because the studies are not needed emergently. Both MRI and BS are available outpatient services. Patients should be immobilized with a thumb spica splint and follow-up should be recommended for either repeat examination or further radiographic testing.

References

1. Fowler, C., Sullivan, B., Williams, L.A., *et al.* (1998) A comparison of bone scintigraphy and MRI in the early diagnosis of the occult scaphoid wrist fracture. *Skeletal Radiology* **27**: 683–687.
2. Kitsis, C., Taylor, M., Chandey, J., *et al.* (1998) Imaging the problem scaphoid. *Injury* **29**(7): 515–520.

Chapter 14 **Blunt Chest Trauma**

Highlights

- Potential injuries in blunt chest trauma include cardiac contusion, pneumothorax, hemothorax, lung contusion, diaphragmatic injury, and injuries to the thoracic aorta.
- No formal decision rules have been validated to identify patients who are at low risk for injuries; however, the findings of chest wall tenderness and hypoxia are highly sensitive for injuries.
- Chest computed tomography (CT) identifies more injuries and should be used in the setting of severely injured patients.
- Data on the use of troponin in detecting cardiac contusion is inconclusive with some studies reporting high sensitivity but one study reports a very low sensitivity (23%).
- Minor cardiac contusions, while detectable using troponin, electrocardiogram (ECG) and echocardiography, are associated with no adverse consequences.

Background

Patients with blunt chest trauma in the emergency department (ED) often require diagnostic testing to exclude potential injuries such as cardiac contusion, pneumothorax, hemothorax, lung contusion, diaphragmatic injuries and injuries to the thoracic aorta. For patients with severe thoracic trauma, gold standard testing (i.e. CT angiography) is often undertaken because in 70–90% multiple injuries are present.

There is a clinical divide between the ambulatory ED patient with a history of blunt chest trauma and chest pain and the multi-injured trauma patient

---

Evidence-Based Emergency Care: Diagnostic Testing and Clinical Decision Rules. By J.M. Pines and W.W. Everett. Published 2008 by Blackwell Publishing, ISBN: 978-14051-5400-0.

because the probability of clinically significant injury is considerably different. Both patient groups are traditionally screened initially with chest radiography (Fig. 14.1). When a patient is ambulatory or not severely injured, they can receive an upright posterior-anterior chest X-ray. By comparison, traditionally in the multi- or severely-injured patient, the initial diagnostic test is a supine anterior-posterior chest X-ray because these patients cannot safely receive upright X-rays. In cases of severe chest trauma, most if not all will receive CT scans of the chest (Fig. 14.2). The initial screening supine X-ray is less sensitive than an upright chest X-ray for detecting thoracic injuries. However, both can be useful in guiding initial management in terms of detecting thoracic injuries in the case of the multi-injured patient, or deciding upon a screening test in patients with minor injuries.

Clinical question one

"Which ED patients need diagnostic chest X-rays following blunt chest trauma?"

A recent pilot study investigated ED patients with blunt chest trauma to predict intrathoracic injuries enrolled 507 patients with blunt chest trauma.[1] The purpose was to use the results as the basis for the derivation of a clinical decision rule to identify patients at low risk for intrathoracic injuries following blunt chest trauma. However, to date there has been no validation of this data as a clinical decision rule. The authors excluded patients less than 15 years old and those with penetrating trauma, isolated head trauma, or a Glasgow Coma Scale score below 14, and those for whom the trauma had occurred more than 72 hours before presentation. Providers filled out surveys prior to viewing radiographic results and documented the mechanism of injury and vital signs including oxygen saturation, patient symptoms, intoxication, distracting injuries, and the presence of visible chest wall injury, chest palpation tenderness, pain on lateral chest compression, crepitus, and abnormal chest auscultation. Significant intrathoracic injuries were defined as pneumothoraces, hemothoraces, aortic injuries, two or more rib fractures, sternal fractures, or pulmonary contusions on blinded plain chest radiography. The prevalence of significant intrathoracic injury was 6% (31 of 492 who had complete data). Tenderness to palpation and chest pain had the highest sensitivity as individual criteria to predict significant injuries (90%), and hypoxia was the most specific (97%). The combination of tenderness to palpation and hypoxia identified all significant injuries: sensitivity 100% (95% CI: 91–100); specificity 50% (95% CI: 45–54); positive predictive value 12% (95% CI: 9–17); and negative predictive value 100% (95% CI: 99–100).

Clinical question two

"How does a chest X-ray compare to a CT scan in excluding thoracic injury in patients with blunt chest trauma?"

Most studies addressing this question have been small and retrospective, involving trauma registries investigating severely injured trauma patients.

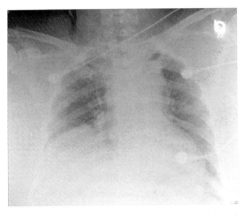

Figure 14.1 Chest X-ray from a patient with a traumatic aortic injury demonstrating a wide mediastinum and blurring of the aortic arch, suggestive of an acute aortic injury.

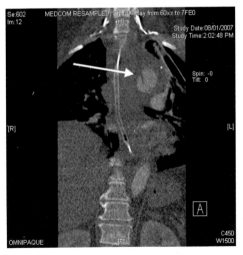

Figure 14.2 A chest computed tomography (CT) was performed on the patient from Figure 14.1 and reconstructions demonstrate a traumatic tear in the aorta (arrow) with a surrounding hematoma.

One study of 112 patients with blunt chest trauma found that four of the nine patients with acute aortic rupture had a normal mediastinum on the initial supine chest X-ray, while helical CT scanning was diagnostic in eight out of the nine, and suggestive in one patient who had a brachiocephalic injury.[2] A recent study from Australia involved a two-year retrospective survey of 141 patients with an injury severity score (ISS) of greater than 15 (i.e. multi-injured trauma patients) and blunt trauma to the chest.[3] Patients had both a supine chest X-ray and a CT of the chest. In patients with chest wall tenderness they found that the CT chest X-ray was more likely to provide further diagnostic information compared to a plain radiography (odds ratio, OR: 6.7; 95% CI: 2.6–17.7). In patients with reduced air entry, the CT was more likely to add clinical information (OR: 4.5; 95% CI: 1.3–15.0), and similarly in patients with an abnormal respiratory effort (OR: 4.1; 95% CI: 1.3–12.7). They also found that a CT scan was more effective than a routine chest X-ray in detecting lung contusions, pneumothoraces, mediastinal, hematomas, as well as fractures (ribs, scapula, sternum and vertebrae).

A prospective study of 103 patients with chest trauma and a mean ISS of 30 (severely injured trauma patients) found that in 67 patients (65%), CT scanning detected major chest trauma complications that were missed on chest X-rays; of those 33 were lung contusions, 27 were pneumothoraces, seven were residual pneumothoraces after chest tube placement, 21 were hemothoraces, five were displaced chest tubes, two patients had diaphragmatic ruptures, and one had a myocardial rupture.[4] In 11 patients, minor additional findings (dystelectasis, small pleural effusion) were visualized on CT scans, and in only 14 patients did chest X-rays and CT scans show the same results.

Another study followed 93 consecutive trauma patients with blunt chest trauma, all of which had anterior-posterior chest radiographs and helical chest CTs.[5] Chest radiography was abnormal in 73% of patients. In 13 of the 25 patients with normal chest radiography (52%), chest CTs demonstrated multiple injuries including two aortic lacerations and one pericardial effusion.

Clinical question three

"What is the role of troponin in excluding myocardial injury in blunt chest trauma?"

Patients with blunt chest trauma can sustain myocardial injuries. In severe cases, this can be dramatic, involving hemodynamic instability. In minor cases, however, blunt cardiac injury can be an occult event because it can produce mild symptoms that may be attributed to the musculoskeletal trauma. Plain radiography (CT and X-ray) is often not helpful in diagnosing cardiac contusions unless there is an associated great vessel or other intrathoracic injury. Laboratory testing, ECG, and echocardiogram are often used to detect injuries. Creatine kinase (CK) levels can be used; however, the detection of cardiac injury in patients with blunt chest trauma can be difficult because levels of the isoenzyme CK-MB can be elevated as a result of skeletal muscle injury.

Troponin I has emerged as a potential indicator of cardiac contusion. One study followed 44 patients with blunt chest trauma and suspected cardiac contusion.[6] Patients underwent serial echocardiograms and troponin I testing. Six out of 44 (14%) had evidence of cardiac injury by echocardiography and all had elevations of CK-MB and troponin I. One patient had elevations of both CK-MB and troponin I and was found to have a pericardial effusion.

Another study followed 32 patients admitted with signs of acute blunt chest trauma.[7] All patients underwent transesophageal echocardiography within 24 hours of injury and had serial troponin I measurements taken. A total of 17 (53%) of patients had abnormal troponin I (>0.4 ng/mL) levels, and 10 had levels of greater than 1 ng/mL. In six out of the ten with troponin, levels exceeding 1 ng/mL, there were segmental wall motion abnormalities consistent with myocardial contusion. None of the patients with troponin levels between 0.4 and 1 ng/mL had abnormal echocardiograms.

Another study followed 96 patients with blunt chest trauma that were admitted to a trauma center for evaluation.[8] A total of 24 out of 96 (28%) had myocardial contusion diagnosed by echocardiogram (12), ECG (29), or both. Notably, all patients survived admission to hospital and were hemodynamically stable. No patients died or had severe in-hospital cardiac complications. There were no differences in the percentage of patients with an elevated CK ratio (CK-MB/total CK) or CK-MB mass concentration among patients with and without cardiac contusion. In patients with cardiac contusion, the percentage of patients with elevated circulating troponin I and troponin T (defined as ≥0.1 μg/L) was higher (23% vs. 3%) In terms of predicting a myocardial contusion in blunt trauma patients, the respective sensitivity, specificity, and negative and positive predictive values were 23, 97, 77, and 75%, respectively, for troponin I, and 12, 100, 74, and 100%, respectively, for tropinin T. The patients were followed for up to 18 months and 88% had complete follow-up. There were no deaths from cardiac complications and none of the patients had any long-term cardiac complications or myocardial failures related to blunt chest trauma.

Comment

The studies on blunt chest trauma reviewed here have considerable methodological issues. Most have very small sample sizes and are retrospective. To date, there is no validated decision rule to identify patients who need radiography, nor are there large studies to differentiate patients who require chest X-rays as opposed to CT scans. Through this review, however, it appears that a number of clinical themes have emerged. For example, in ED patients with blunt chest trauma the prevalence of clinically significant injuries is relatively low (6%) and clinical factors, such as the presence of tenderness to palpation and chest pain, may suggest the need for chest radiography. In patients with severe chest trauma or a high index of suspicion for intrathoracic injury, CT scans seem to be the study of choice given the potential for missed injuries on initial chest X-rays, especially given the high miss rate (50%) in severely injured patients.

The data on myocardial contusion seems to be inconclusive. While some studies have reported that troponin I is a sensitive marker for myocardial injury, one study found that the sensitivity was only 23%. An interesting finding was that in patients with minor contusions (without any hemodynamic instability) no patients had any clinical complications, indicating that the contusion, although detectable radiographically or by ECG, was not clinically significant. Certainly a larger study is needed before concluding that objective findings such as these are clinically benign.

References

1. Rodriguez, R.M., Hendey, G.M., Marek, G., et al. (2006) A pilot study to derive clinical variables for selective chest radiography in blunt trauma patients. *Annals of Emergency Medicine* **47**: 415–418.
2. Demetriades, D., Gomez, H., Velmahos, G.C., et al. (1998) Routine helical computed tomographic evaluation of the mediastinum in high-risk blunt trauma patients. *Archives of Surgery* **133**: 1084–1088.
3. Traub, M., Stevenson, M., McEvoy, S., et al. (2007) The use of chest computed tomography versus chest X-ray in patients with major blunt trauma. *Injury* **38**: 43–7.
4. Trupka, A., Waydas, C., Hallfeldt, K.K., et al. (1997) Value of thoracic computed tomography in the first assessment of severely injured patients with blunt chest trauma: results of a prospective study. *Journal of Trauma* **43**: 405–411.
5. Exadaktylos, A.K., Sclabas, G. and Schmid, S.W. (2001) Do we really need routine computed tomographic scanning in the primary evaluation of blunt chest trauma in patients with "normal" chest radiograph? *Journal of Trauma* **51**: 1173–1176.
6. Adams, J.E., Davila-Roman, V.G., Bessey, P.Q., et al. (1996) Improved detection of cardiac contusion with cardiac troponin I. *American Heart Journal* **131**(2): 308–312.

7. Mori, F., Zuppiroli, A., Ognibene, A., *et al.* (2001) Cardiac contusion in blunt chest trauma: a combined study of transesophageal echocardiography and cardiac troponin I determination. *Italian Heart Journal* **2**: 222–227.
8. Bertinchant, J.P., Polge, A., Mohty, D., *et al.* (2000) Evaluation of incidence, clinical significance, and prognostic value of circulating cardiac troponin I and T elevation in hemodynamically stable patients with suspected myocardial contusion after blunt chest trauma. *Journal of Trauma* **48**: 924–931.

Chapter 15 **Occult Hip Fracture**

Highlights

- Hip fractures will not be seen on initial plain X-rays in nearly 10% of patients with hip pain after falls or trauma.
- Advanced imaging, either with computed tomography (CT) or magnetic resonance imaging (MRI), should be used in cases of suspected occult fracture.

Background

Hip fractures are common in the elderly population, with an incidence rate of approximately 250 000 per year. A large proportion of patients with hip fracture will present to the emergency department (ED) for evaluation and treatment, typically following a fall or an acute traumatic injury. The diagnosis of hip fracture is normally not a diagnostic dilemma because plain radiographs are often confirmatory studies, particularly in patients with classic anatomic deformities (Fig. 15.1). However, a small proportion of patients with hip fracture (2–9%) will initially have negative plain films. These 'occult' hip fractures are more common in the elderly because of the high prevalence of osteoporosis. A diagnostic dilemma comes when there is a high clinical likelihood of hip fracture based on physical examination or history, and when plain radiographs are either negative or equivocal. The classic case is an older adult patient who has fallen, has hip tenderness, and can not bear any weight on the affected leg. A missed diagnosis of hip fracture can place elderly patients at substantial risk of displacement, avascular necrosis, and subsequently, for more involved surgical procedures.

Evidence-Based Emergency Care: Diagnostic Testing and Clinical Decision Rules. By J.M. Pines and W.W. Everett. Published 2008 by Blackwell Publishing, ISBN: 978-14051-5400-0.

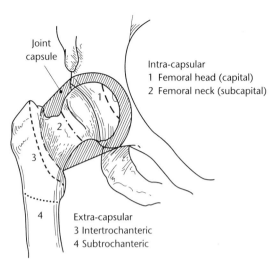

Figure 15.1 Hip fractures. This illustration depicts the different types of proximal femoral fractures. (Source: Knoop *et al. Atlas of Emergency Medicine* 2nd Edition © 2002. Reproduced with permission of The McGraw-Hill Companies.)

An approach to the diagnosis of occult hip fractures has evolved over the past 10 years. Previously, repeat plain films or bone scans had been advocated. Bone scans will typically become positive 24 to 72 hours following an acute fracture. Patients who present to the ED with acute traumatic hip pain and who are unable to ambulate require further imaging to exclude occult hip fracture. The primary dilemma for the emergency physician is therefore whether to order a CT scan of the hip or an MRI.

Clinical question

"Which is the optimal diagnostic modality when pursuing the diagnosis of occult hip fracture in the ED?"
Since bone scanning can take days to become positive and serial plain films are not typically performed in the ED setting, we believe that these modalities are impractical as sensitive, rapid detection strategies for occult hip fracture. While there are cases series and retrospective studies that address this question indirectly, there are very few studies investigating whether a CT or MRI should be ordered.[1] The literature primarily describes cases where MRI has been used to diagnose hip fractures, and cases reporting a negative CT followed by a positive MRI for fracture. The concern is that CT scans can miss very small impacted fractures of the femoral head and non-displaced

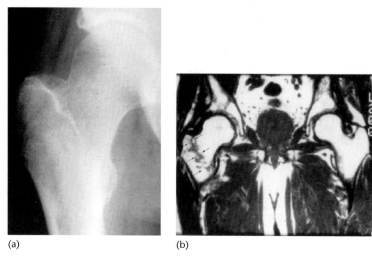

(a)   (b)

Figure 15.2 Occult hip fracture. (a) Anteroposterior radiograph of a 55-year-old
patient on steroids who had right hip pain after a fall. No fracture is evident. (b) T1-
weighted coronal magnetic resonance scan of the same hip clearly demonstrates a
nondisplaced intertrochanteric femoral shaft fracture (*arrows*). (Reproduced from
Tintinalli *et al.* (2004) *Tintinalli's Emergency Medicine: A Comprehensive Study Guide*
6th Edition, with permission of The McGraw-Hill Companies.)

fractures that run parallel to the axial plane.[2] One study assessed 13 elderly
patients that had suffered a fall and that had no evidence of a fracture on plain
films.[3] A total of six patients underwent CT and MRI, and seven underwent
MRI only. In the six patients that had both studies, four of the CT images
resulted in misdiagnosis due to inaccuracy. While this is a very small study, it
demonstrates that MRI is likely to be more sensitive than CT scanning when
evaluating patients with occult hip fracture. In the group that had MRI only,
all seven patients received an accurate diagnosis of hip fracture.

A recent retrospective study sought to determine the prevalence of hip
and pelvic fractures in ED patients with hip pain and negative initial radiographs.[4] This was a retrospective study where plain films and MRIs were
ordered at the discretion of the treating physician. A structured follow-up
of 85% of the patients was conducted one month after the visit. Of the
545 patients who had negative initial radiographs, 11% underwent hip MRI
during the ED visit and this identified 24 additional patients with hip fractures with good interobserver agreement among radiologists (Fig. 15.2). There
were no patients in the one-month follow-up period that subsequently had
hip fractures identified.

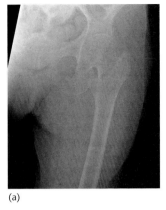
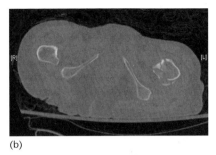

(a)   (b)

Figure 15.3 Intertrochanteric fracture was suspected on the left hip plain X-ray (a), and was confirmed with the noncontrast CT scan (b).

Comment

While are few reports in the literature that directly address whether CT or MRI is the optimal diagnostic test for investigating occult hip fractures, case series and retrospective studies support the use of MRI for this purpose. In fact, MRI is currently recognized as the gold standard for diagnosing hip fractures based on reported cases of negative CTs and positive MRIs. Additionally, the absence of any subsequent diagnoses of hip fracture over a one one-month follow-up in patients with negative MRIs in one study supports the belief that this modality is close to 100% sensitive for fractures. However, MRI may not be available at all EDs, particularly during off-hours. Individual patient and hospital circumstances should dictate whether a CT should be ordered first because CTs can occasionally diagnose hip fractures that are not present on plain radiographs (Fig. 15.3). In situations where the plain films and the CT are negative for fracture and there is still a high clinical likelihood, then MRI should be ordered or the patient should be admitted for MRI, if it is not readily available in the ED.

References

1. Mlinek, E.J., Clark, K.C. and Walker, C. (1998) Limited magnetic resonance imaging in the diagnosis of occult hip fracture. *American Journal of Emergency Medicine* **16**: 390–393.
2. Perron, A.D., Miller, M.D. and Brady, W.J. (2002) Orthopedic pitfalls in the ED: Radiographically occult hip fracture. *American Journal of Emergency Medicine* **20**: 234–237.

3. Lubovsky, O., Liebergall, M., Mattan, Y., *et al.* (2005) Early diagnosis of hip fractures: MRI versus CT scan. *Injury* **36**: 788–792.
4. Dominguez, S., Liu, P., Roberts, C., *et al.* (2005) Prevalence of traumatic hip and pelvic fractures in patients with suspected hip fracture and negative initial standard radiographs – a study of emergency department patients. *Academic Emergency Medicine* **12**: 366–369.

SECTION 3
Cardiology

Chapter 16 **Heart Failure**

Highlights

- The incidence of heart failure is high with nearly half a million new cases annually in the US.
- Differentiating acute heart failure from chronic obstructive pulmonary disease (COPD) or severe asthma is sometimes a challenge in the emergency department (ED).
- Clinical impression is sensitive but nonspecific for heart failure, while an S3 heart sound and chest X-ray findings suggestive of heart failure are specific but not sensitive.
- Elevated brain natriuretic peptide (BNP) levels can be informative, but are not a definitive test for heart failure.

Background

Heart failure is a widespread disease that accounts for more than one million hospitalizations annually in the US, with nearly half a million new cases arising annually. Multiple models of the various pathophysiologic paradigms of the cardiac decompensation process have been described and include cardiorenal and cardiocirculatory models, and neurohormonal levels.[1] Briefly, the cardiorenal model describes heart failure as a process of peripheral edema resulting from decreased renal blood flow, which in turn is a result of cardiac dysfunction. The cardiocirculatory model is based on a cascade of events starting with peripheral vasoconstriction resulting in reduced preload, ventricular wall stress, and arterial vasoconstriction leading to an increased afterload. In turn, cardiac output drops and renal perfusion decreases resulting in sodium retention and edema. Finally, the neurohormonal model

Evidence-Based Emergency Care: Diagnostic Testing and Clinical Decision Rules. By J.M. Pines and W.W. Everett. Published 2008 by Blackwell Publishing, ISBN: 978-14051-5400-0.

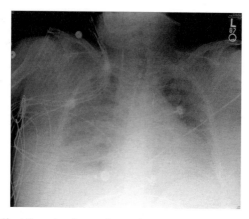

Figure 16.1 Chest X-ray showing cardiomegaly, prominent vascular markings, and interstitial edema, consistent with congestive heart failure.

acknowledges the role that neurohormones play when there is decreased cardiac function, increased vascular tone, and fluctuating volume retention elements, all of which are found to some degree in most patients with heart failure.

Heart failure is conceptually a syndrome with multiple possible etiologies that manifests clinically in a spectrum of signs and symptoms. Given the complex nature of the disease, we are challenged to use what is immediately available to us—the patient's history and physical findings—and, when possible, diagnostic tests to confirm the diagnosis. However, an exhaustive evaluation is not always possible and we must often begin treatment while the workup is getting started. The most common presentation of heart failure is a patient with new or progressive dyspnea, and the sensation of difficulty or increased effort in breathing. Indeed, most of us confronted with the dyspneic patient contemplate the diagnosis of heart failure versus primary pulmonary processes such as COPD or severe asthma. This review will focus on physical examination findings, including the presence of an S3 (ventricular filling gallop), routine chest X-ray results, and BNP levels, that may be used to confirm or rule out the diagnosis of heart failure.

Clinical question

"Are the physical examination findings of an S3, chest X-ray, or BNP analysis sufficiently predictive in establishing or excluding the diagnosis of heart failure in an acutely dyspneic patient?"

A meta-analysis in 2005 examined the accuracy of multiple factors (history, physical, diagnostic studies) in making the diagnosis of heart failure among ED patients with acute dyspnea.[2] The pooled analysis examined only studies with original data in which patients were aged 18 years or older, and in which there was a reference standard that included a panel of physician reviewers that examined clinical data and cardiac studies to determine if the patient had heart failure. Studies were excluded if they were population-based or review articles, used only echocardiography or computed tomography (CT) scans as a reference standard, did not report clinical examination data, or did not specifically state that patients with dyspnea were enrolled. Out of a total of 815 citations, 18 studies were included in the analysis.

Overall, clinical impression was moderately specific (86%) as a diagnostic tool, but insensitive (61%). The average likelihood ratios for the diagnosis of heart failure were LR+ 4.4 (95% CI: 1.8–10) and LR– 0.45 (95% CI: 0.28–0.73). When considering specifically patients that had a history of asthma or COPD the performance characteristics for overall clinical impression were 37% for sensitivity and 96% for specificity, and corresponding pooled likelihood ratios were LR+ 9.9 (95% CI: 5.3–18) and LR– 0.65 (95% CI: 0.55–0.77).

The presence of a third heart sound was highly specific (99%) in the diagnosis of heart failure but not sensitive (13%), with corresponding pooled likelihood ratios of LR+ 11.0 (95% CI: 4.9–25) and LR– 0.88 (95% CI: 0.83–0.94). Among patients with a specific history of asthma or COPD, sensitivity was 17% and specificity 100%, and corresponding pooled likelihood ratios were LR 57+ (95% CI: 7.6–425) and LR– 0.83 (95% CI: 0.75–0.91).

Chest X-rays that revealed pulmonary vascular congestion and interstitial edema (Fig. 16.1) were highly specific (96% and 97%, respectively), but neither were found to be sensitive (54% and 34%, respectively). Both were associated with very high LR+ and low LR– values: for pulmonary vascular congestion LR+ was 12.0 (95% CI: 6.8–21) and LR– was 0.48 (95% CI: 0.28–0.83), and for interstitial edema LR+ was 12.0 (95% CI: 5.2–27) and LR– was 0.68 (95% CI: 0.54–0.85).

BNP is a neurohormone that is secreted by cardiac ventricles under conditions of increased ventricular volume and pressure. An international, multicenter, prospective study examined ED patients with acute dyspnea to investigate the use of BNP as a marker for congestive heart failure.[3] Clinical data was collected and blood samples were obtained for analysis. Patients with a history of myocardial infarction or advanced renal failure were excluded due to the fact that BNP levels are known to be elevated in these conditions. Patients with blunt or penetrating chest trauma or the presence of a pneumothorax were also excluded. The final determination of heart failure was made by two cardiologists who were blinded to the BNP levels. A history of heart failure, reported by patients, was dichotomized into acute exacerbations of heart failure or dyspnea from non-heart failure causes. A total of 1586 patients were enrolled and a total of 744 patients had a final diagnosis of heart failure (47%). Dyspnea not related to heart failure was recorded in 72 patients (5%). Table 16.1 shows the BNP levels for each group of patients. Table 16.2 demonstrates increasing levels of BNP in the higher classes, assigned according to the New York Heart Association (NYHA) functional classification system.

A BNP level ≥100 pg/mL was independently associated with heart failure [odds ratio (OR) 29.6 (95% CI: 18–49)]. Using a cutoff of 100 pg/mL the BNP assay had a sensitivity of 90% (95% CI: 88–92), specificity of 76% (95% CI: 73–79), positive predictive value (PPV) of 79% (95% CI: 76–81), negative predictive value (NPV) of 89% (95% CI: 87–91), and an accuracy of 83%. Other factors that were found to be strongly and independently associated with heart failure were a history of heart failure (OR 11.0 [95% CI: 7–19]), and cephalization of vessels on chest X-rays [OR 11.0 (95% CI: 5–21)]. Interestingly, an S3 was not associated with heart failure in this large study.

A subset analysis of the Breathing Not Right Multinational Study examined the accuracy of the chest radiograph in diagnosing heart failure.[4] Eight-hundred and eighty patients with complete data were included and heart failure was the final diagnosis in 51% of patients. Assessments of the chest radiographs were performed by radiologists who were blinded to clinical

Table 16.1 Brain natriuretic peptide (BNP) levels in emergency department patients with acute dyspnea from Maisel et al.[3]

	No heart failure (n = 770)	Non-heart failure dyspnea (n = 72)	Heart failure (n = 744)
BNP, pg/mL (± SD)	110 (225)	346 (390)	675 (450)

Table 16.2 Brain natriuretic peptide (BNP) levels and the extent of heart failure, according to the New York Heart Academy (NYHA) functional classification from Maisel et al.[3]

	NYHA functional classification			
	I	II	III	IV
BNP, pg/mL (± SD)	244 (286)	389 (374)	640 (447)	817 (435)

Table 16.3 Diagnostic performance of variables used for predicting heart failure from Knudsen et al.[4]

	Odds ratio (95% CI)	Sensitivity %	Specificity %	LR+	LR−
CXR findings					
Alveolar edema	7.1 (2.5–20.6)	6	99	7.0	1.0
Cephalization	15.4 (9.4–25.3)	41	96	9.4	0.6
Cardiomegaly	15.4 (11.1–21.3)	79	80	4.0	0.3
Interstitial edema	17.1 (8.6–34.2)	27	98	12.7	0.7
Clinical findings					
S3	9.1 (4.1–20)	13	98	8.1	0.9

CXR, chest X-ray.

findings. Specific chest radiograph findings of alveolar edema, interstitial edema, alveolar edema, cephalization, and cardiomegaly were present in 4%, 15%, 23%, and 50% of the patients, respectively. The authors also included data on the presence of a third heart sound, which was present in 7% of patients. Table 16.3 shows the univariate performance characteristics of the chest radiograph and S3 findings. Multivariate logistic modeling, performed using all of the clinical, historic, radiographic, and BNP data, found that three chest X-ray findings were significantly associated with a diagnosis of heart failure: interstitial edema had an OR of 7.0 (95% CI: 2.9–17), cephalization had an OR of 6.4 (95% CI: 3.3–12.5), and cardiomegaly had an OR of 2.3 (95% CI: 1.4–3.7).

Collins et al. recently compared physician auscultation of heart sounds with electronically detected heart sounds in order to assess the utility of the third heart sound in diagnosing heart failure.[5] Using a convenience sample of patients in four EDs presenting with signs or symptoms of heart failure, the authors compared prospectively recorded physician determination of the presence/absence of a third heart sound with electronically recorded heart sounds that were analyzed in a blinded fashion after the patient encounter. The final diagnosis of heart failure was made by two senior cardiologists who had copies of the complete patient charts, edited to remove all heart sound and BNP data. The electronic heart sound was taken as the criterion standard in the comparison against physician-determined auscultation for the third heart sound.

A total of 439 patients were enrolled and 343 were included in the final analysis. Excluded patients were either pilot subjects or those for which there were problems in obtaining or interpreting electronic heart sound data. Acute heart failure was the final diagnosis in 133 (39%) patients. Table 16.4

Table 16.4 Test parameters for auscultated and electronically detected S3 in patients with acute heart failure (HF) from Collins *et al.*[5]

	Auscultated			Electronically detected		
	Acute HF (+)	Acute HF (−)	Total	Acute HF (+)	Acute HF (−)	Total
S3 present (+)	21	7	28	45	14	59
S3 absent (−)	107	200	307	88	196	284
Total	128	207	335	133	210	343
Sensitivity, % (95% CI)	16 (11–24)			34 (26–43)		
Specificity, % (95% CI)	97 (93–99)			93 (89–96)		
PPV, % (95% CI)	84 (76–89)			66 (57–74)		
NPV, % (95% CI)	3 (2–7)			7 (4–11)		
Diagnostic accuracy, % (95% CI)	66 (61–71)			70 (65–75)		

NPV, negative predictive value; PPV, positive predictive value.

shows the performance characteristics for both auscultation and electronically detected S3. The test characteristics did not change significantly when patients with a past history of heart failure were excluded.

The limitations of this study included the method of patient enrollment—convenience sampling, which may have resulted in a selection bias. The lack of blinding of the examining physician to the rest of the clinical information and findings could have also lead to biased reporting of auscultated heart sounds.

Comments

The accurate diagnosis of acute heart failure is the primary goal of acute care physicians when evaluating dyspneic patients. Evaluation of the presence of a third heart sound has been repeatedly shown to be highly specific, but lacking in sensitivity. This means that determination of the presence of a third heart sound can yield rapid information for the clinician; in other words, if you detect an S3 in the setting of appropriate clinical presentation, you can predict with moderately high confidence that the patient has acute heart failure. Furthermore, a small study comparing bedside auscultation to electronically recorded and interpreted heart tones indicates that physical examination is reliable. However, physical diagnosis with a reliance on patient interviews and physical examinations should continue to be the bedrock for clinical medicine.

The plain chest radiograph can contribute additional data regarding the likelihood of acute heart failure. Findings of interstitial and alveolar edema, vascular redistribution in the form of cephalization, as well as cardiomegaly, are all highly specific for the diagnosis of acute heart failure. However, the abysmally low sensitivity of these methods should deter the clinician from a total reliance on chest radiography in the setting of a normal or non-diagnostic X-ray.

Elevated BNP levels can further help us to diagnose acute heart failure, especially when presented in conjunction with other features, such as radiographic findings or the presence of an S3. We do though offer a word of caution about the use of BNP as a diagnostic marker: conditions that cause an elevation in right-heart pressures in the acute setting (as in acute myocardial infarction, pulmonary embolism) or in the chronic setting (cor pulmonale or pulmonary hypertension), as well as systemic conditions that cause volume overload, as in the case of an end-stage renal disease patient on hemodialysis, can also be associated with elevated BNP levels. Therefore, when using elevated BNP as a diagnostic test for acute heart failure, results should be interpreted with these other conditions listed on the differential diagnosis.

Rapid assessment of the acute dyspneic patient using a solid physical examination, plain chest radiography, and analysis of BNP levels if possible, can assist clinicians in tailoring appropriate therapies for acute heart failure. However, further testing is recommended in order to establish left ventricular function and to rule out proximal causes of acute heart failure, and this should prompt inpatient admissions in most cases.

References

1. Chung, P. and Hermann, L. (2006) Acute decompensated heart failure: formulating an evidence-based approach to diagnosis and treatment (Part 1). *Mount Sinai Journal of Medicine* **73**(2): 506–515.
2. Wang, C.S., FitzGerald, J.M., Schulzer, M., Mak, E. and Ayas, N.T. (2005) Does this dyspneic patient in the emergency department have congestive heart failure? *Journal of the American Medical Association* **294**(15): 1944–1956.
3. Maisel, A.S., Krishnaswamy, P., Nowak, R.M., *et al.* and for the Breathing Not Properly Multinational Study Investigators (2002) Rapid measurement of B-type natriuretic peptide in the emergency diagnosis of heart failure. *New England Journal of Medicine* **347**(3): 161–167.
4. Knudsen, C.W., Omland, T., Clopton, P., *et al.* (2004) Diagnostic value of B-type natriuretic peptide and chest radiographic findings in patients with acute dyspnea. *American Journal of Medicine* **116**: 363–368.
5. Collins, S.P., Lindsell, C.J., Peacock, W.F., *et al.* (2006) The combined utility of an S3 heart sound and B-type natriuretic peptide levels in emergency department patients with dyspnea. *Journal of Cardiac Failure* **12**(4): 286–292.

Chapter 17 **Syncope**

Highlights

- Patients with syncope can appear clinically benign in the emergency department (ED), but a small proportion will have life-threatening conditions.
- The San Francisco syncope rule has been derived and validated for identifying patients at a high risk of serious outcomes, and can help risk stratify patients with syncope.
- Because the San Francisco syncope rule was shown to be insensitive in an external validation study, it cannot be recommended at this time as a definitive guide for admission decisions.

Background

Syncope is a transient loss of consciousness associated with a return to pre-existing neurological function and accounts for up to 3% of all ED visits. Syncope is a symptom that has a wide variety of causes, ranging from the benign to the life-threatening. The evaluation of syncope poses a diagnostic challenge to the emergency physician because in up to 50% of cases the cause for syncope is unclear, even after a thorough ED evaluation. The potential for serious causes of syncope include cardiac arrhythmias, myocardial infarction, ruptured ectopic pregnancy, stroke, subarachnoid hemorrhage, and pulmonary embolism.

As a result of the diagnostic uncertainty and the multiple potentially serious etiologies of syncope, patients are frequently admitted to the hospital for further evaluation. As an inpatient, a patient may receive further diagnostic testing such as an echocardiogram or electroencephalogram, or may undergo

Evidence-Based Emergency Care: Diagnostic Testing and Clinical Decision Rules. By J.M. Pines and W.W. Everett. Published 2008 by Blackwell Publishing, ISBN: 978-14051-5400-0.

cardiac monitoring and cardiac stress testing. Specific treatments, such as pacemakers or defibrillators, can be used if a cardiac arrhythmia is determined as the cause for syncope, or changes in medication may be made to reduce the risk of syncope in the future.

Over the past 10 years multiple studies have been performed to identify patients with syncope who may be safe for discharge after ED evaluation. Most recently, a decision rule to identify low-risk patients with syncope was derived and validated and has been named the San Francisco syncope rule.

Clinical question

"Does the San Francisco rule reliably identify low-risk patients with syncope who are safe for hospital discharge after ED evaluation?"

Initial studies of the diagnosis and prognosis of syncope attempted to identify ED patients with syncope who were at risk for poor outcomes such as death, myocardial infarction and arrhythmias, in order to provide a framework for risk stratification. In 1997, Martin *et al.* performed a prospective analysis of patients who presented to the ED with syncope to determine risk factors for arrhythmias and sudden death at one year.[1] They included two cohorts: a derivation cohort for which data was collected between March 1981 and February 1984, and a validation cohort for which data was collected between August 1987 and February 1991. Because of the long time period over which the study data was gathered, there were differences in data collection strategies and in the evaluation between the derivation and validation cohorts. All patients underwent a standard syncope evaluation including electrocardiogram (ECG), routine laboratory testing, and in excess of 24 hours of cardiac monitoring. The primary outcomes in the study were arrhythmias (broadly defined) and mortality at one year. The authors found that significant multivariable predictors for one-year mortality included: abnormal ECG, a history of ventricular arrhythmia and/or congestive heart failure, age above 45 years, and being of non-white race. For mortality, an additional significant risk factor was having no prior history of syncope. When applied to the validation cohort, these risk factors and combinations thereof were used in an overall risk score that totaled the number of risk factors; this performed fairly well, despite there being a lower event rate in the validation cohort. The authors also looked at cardiac mortality and found that in the absence of any of these risk factors the overall mortality from cardiac causes approached zero. Some of the limitations of the study included the fact that the study was performed at one center and that electrophysiological testing was not performed on all patients.

Another study to investigate risk stratification of patients with syncope, derived and validated in Italy, is called the OESIL (Osservatorio Epidemiologico sulla Sincope nel Lazio) risk score.[2] The investigators used a similar method to that of Martin et al.[1] and followed patients who presented to the ED with syncope to determine risk factors for mortality at one year. Their inclusion criteria were broadened to include patients as young as 12 years old. The authors identified the following as significant univariable predictors of mortality: age above 65 years, hypertension, a clinical history of cardiovascular disease, diabetes, syncope without prodrome, syncope-related traumatic injuries, and an abnormal ECG. In multivariable analysis the following predictors were all found to be significant and these were combined to form the OESIL risk score where each factor was given one point: (i) age above 65 years; (ii) a history of cardiovascular disease; (iii) syncope without prodrome; and (iv) an abnormal ECG. Patients who presented with zero or one point had a mortality rate near zero at one year. From this the authors concluded that these patients were low risk. However, the authors did not measure interventions such as the fitting of pacemakers or defibrillators, or any further diagnostic testing that was performed on these patients.

More recently, Quinn et al. performed a derivation study and validated the use of the San Francisco syncope rule.[3] In comparison to previous studies, the authors used outcome at seven days to determine whether a patient with syncope required hospital admission. The authors prospectively followed 684 patients with syncope or near syncope that were evaluated in the ED. Physicians filled out a structured data form for each patient and serious outcomes (death, myocardial infarction, arrhythmia, pulmonary embolism, stroke, subarachnoid hemorrhage, significant hemorrhage, or return to the ED) were recorded at seven days after ED arrival. There were 79 serious outcomes in the derivation database. Individual chi-square tests (test of association for categorical variables) were performed for predictor variables and serious outcomes. They also performed a kappa analysis (test of inter-rater agreement) and only used variables with good agreement (0.5–1) for the decision rule. The goal, as in all decision rules, was to approach 100% sensitivity and to maximize specificity as much as possible.

The absence of all of the following risk-factors was 96% sensitive and 62% specific for identifying serious outcomes at seven days:
- an abnormal ECG;
- a complaint of shortness of breath;
- a hematocrit of less than 30%;
- a triage systolic blood pressure of less than 90 mmHg; and
- a history of congestive heart failure.

The authors reported that when applied to the derivation cohort, this could have potentially decreased the admission rate for syncope by 10%.

The validation of the San Francisco syncope rule included 791 consecutive ED visits and there were 53 serious reported outcomes.[4] The authors found that the rule was 98% sensitive (95% CI: 89–100) and 56% specific (95% CI: 52–60). Some limitations of the study included the fact that the participants were all from one hospital. Because the authors used a composite outcome that included multiple serious outcomes, the study was not powered to detect any one outcome (such as pulmonary embolism) individually. The authors refrained from stating that the San Francisco syncope rule was a definitive guide for which patients should necessarily be admitted, stating rather that it should be used more as a risk stratification rule and citing the fact that there are many reasons for hospital admission.

Another group performed an independent validation of the San Francisco syncope rule in an ED population in a single academic center.[5] At the time of care, physicians recorded the elements of the rule and they then contacted patients at 14 days with a structured interview. The primary outcome of the study was the sensitivity of the San Francisco syncope rule for predicting serious events at seven days. A secondary outcome of the study was the prediction of any serious clinical events that were not detected during the initial ED visit. They consented 477 patients and obtained full records (either from the admission or through telephone follow-up). The serious event prevalence was 12%, and 3% had a serious diagnosis that was not identified during the initial ED evaluation. They reported a sensitivity of 89% (95% CI: 81–97) and a specificity of 42% (95% CI: 37–48) for the San Francisco syncope rule in predicting seven-day serious outcomes. They also reported a sensitivity of 69% (95% CI: 46–95) and 42% (95% CI: 37–48) for a serious diagnosis that was not identified during the initial ED evaluation. The authors concluded that the San Francisco syncope rule had a lower sensitivity and specificity than had been previously reported.

Comment

While the San Francisco syncope rule does provide a good risk stratification scheme for determining which patients are at a low risk for serious short-term outcomes, it does not provide us with a definitive guide for determining which patients should be admitted or discharged. While it was validated in a similar population to that from which it was derived, when tested on an external ED population it did not perform well. Because syncope is a symptom with heterogeneous causes, to power a study to rule out the presence or absence of any specific cause would require a large number of patients.

In the context of relevant ED risk stratification, the San Francisco syncope rule comes closer than previous studies that had considered one-year mortality. From a patient perspective, one-year mortality is certainly important and determining which patients are high risk can guide decisions on whether to admit, and whether to obtain further testing and follow the patients longitudinally. When we evaluated ED patients with syncope, our evaluation considered immediate life threats and whether the cause of syncope required emergency admission for further testing and/or treatment for the primary cause.

So, this leaves us with the question of whether to use or not to use the San Francisco syncope rule. While one study has suggested that the rule does not work, we would recommend using it as a risk stratification tool and to inform decisions regarding whether to admit patients with syncope, but certainly not as a definitive guide for admission decisions.

References

1. Martin, T.P., Hanusa, B.H. and Kapoor, W.N. (1997) Risk stratification of patients with syncope. *Annals of Emergency Medicine* **29**: 459–466.
2. Colivicchi, F., Ammirati, F., Melina, D., *et al.* (2003) Development and prospective validation of a risk stratification system for patients with syncope in the emergency department: the OESIL risk score *European Heart Journal* **24**: 811–819.
3. Quinn, J.V., Steill, I.G., McDermott, D.A., *et al.* (2004) Derivation of the San Francisco syncope rule to predict patients with short-term serious outcomes. *Annals of Emergency Medicine* **43**: 224–232.
4. Quinn, J., McDermott, D., Stiell, I., *et al.* (2006) Prospective validation of the San Francisco syncope rule to predict patients with serious outcomes. *Annals of Emergency Medicine* **47**: 448–454.
5. Sun, B.C., Mangione, C.M., Merchant, G., *et al.* (2007) External validation of the San Francisco syncope rule. *Annals of Emergency Medicine* **49**: 420–427.

Chapter 18 **Acute Coronary Syndrome**

Highlights

- Acute coronary syndrome is a spectrum of conditions ranging from acute myocardial infarction to stable angina.
- Troponin I is poorly sensitive but highly specific for initial testing, but sensitivity increases considerably with serial testing.
- Any positive troponin I test is predictive of higher short-term risks for adverse outcomes.
- Non-invasive stress testing can determine the presence and extent of coronary disease.
- Exercise electrocardiogram (ECG) stress testing is widely available but lacks sensitivity or specificity.
- Pharmacologic agents can increase sensitivity when combined with myocardial perfusion imaging, and when combined with echocardiography the specificity is maximized.
- Stress echocardiography with dobutamine has higher specificity in women compared to nuclear scintigraphy.
- Computed tomography (CT) coronary angiography may be useful for low-risk emergency department (ED) patients and appears to be at least as sensitive and specific as stress myocardial perfusion imaging.

Background

Coronary artery disease (CAD) is one of the main causes of death in the US and worldwide. Patients with symptomatic CAD frequently present directly to the ED with symptoms of acute chest pain. The spectrum of acute chest pain and other symptoms of myocardial ischemia, ranging from acute

Evidence-Based Emergency Care: Diagnostic Testing and Clinical Decision Rules. By J.M. Pines and W.W. Everett. Published 2008 by Blackwell Publishing, ISBN: 978-14051-5400-0.

myocardial infarction (AMI) with myocardial necrosis to reversible ischemic damage or unstable angina (UA), are described clinically by the term acute coronary syndrome (ACS). The first step in ED management of patients is to obtain a 12-lead electrocardiogram (ECG). Findings on the initial ECG may be diagnostic or suggestive of ACS, but sometimes the ECG is normal or non-diagnostic. Distinguishing AMI and UA from other non-cardiac chest pain typically involves serial ECGs and/or serial analysis of serum biomarkers of myocardial injury, in conjunction with diagnostic imaging (stress test or CT scan) or cardiac catheterization.

For patients presenting to the ED with acute chest pain, an ECG should be obtained promptly in order to detect the presence of ST-segment elevation, new left bundle branch blocks, or new dynamic ST changes indicative of AMI. And while the standard ECG is the single best test to identify patients with AMI when they present to the ED, it has relatively low sensitivity for the detection of AMI. In patients with AMI, the ST segment is elevated on the initial ECG in approximately 50% of cases. Because of the insensitivity of ECG, other tests are incorporated into the work-up of patients with acute chest pain with suspected ACS, including analysis of cardiac specific biomarkers and diagnostic imaging or stress testing.

The clinical questions that are likely to arise during the assessment of a patient with suspected ACS are the test characteristics of cardiac biomarkers, non-invasive stress testing, and cardiac CT imaging.

Serum biomarkers

Serum biomarkers have been used in the assessment of ED patients with suspected ACS but with no history of ECG signs of ST-elevation, myocardial infarction, or dynamic ECG changes for over 30 years. Technological advances have meant that the use of nonspecific biomarkers, such as lactose dehydrogenase (LDH) and aspartate aminotransferase (AST) has declined and more sensitive and specific cardiac specific biomarkers, including creatine kinase (CK)-MB, troponin T, and troponin I, are now used routinely. The biokinetic properties of the cardiac troponins are similar in terms of the increase in serum concentrations, usually within 4–6 h of AMI (similar changes are seen in CK-MB); however, the serum levels remain elevated for over a week. Both I and T subunits are part of the striated cardiac muscle contractile unit (Fig. 18.1). The I subunit is a smaller, inhibitory protein and, as it is not found in the serum in the absence of myocardial injury, it should exhibit high sensitivity and specificity. The T subunit is larger and is not found in the serum of patients in the absence of heart complaints or heart disease. It is released into the serum at a slightly slower rate than troponin I and has been

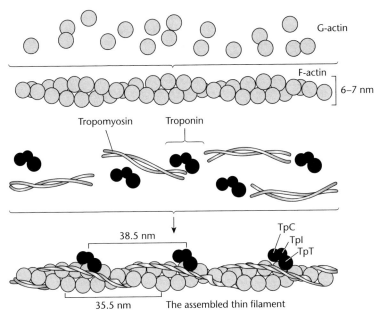

Figure 18.1 Schematic representation of the thin filament, showing the spatial configuration of its three major protein components: actin, myosin, and tropomyosin. The upper panel shows individual molecules of G-actin. The middle panel shows actin monomers assembled into F-actin. Individual molecules of tropomyosin (two strands wound around one another) and troponin (made up of its three subunits) are also shown. The lower panel shows the assembled thin filament, consisting of F-actin, tropomyosin, and the three subunits of troponin (TpC, TpI, and TpT). (Source: Murray *et al. Harper's Illustrated Biochemistry* 25th Edition © 2000. Reproduced with permission of The McGraw-Hill Companies)

found to be elevated in patients with reversible ischemic injury, resulting in a greater number of false positives in the setting of UA.

Clinical question one

"What are the performance characteristics of the cardiac troponins (I and T) in terms of the diagnosis of acute cardiac ischemia? Do these differ when initial biomarker levels are compared to serial biomarkers?"

One systematic review and three meta-analyses have examined the diagnostic performance of biochemical markers for ACS, including AMI and UA. All of these studies were published in 2001 and therefore do not incorporate

Table 18.1 Summary performance characteristics of biomarker studies in the diagnosis of acute myocardial infarction in emergency department (ED) patients from published studies, 1966–1998[1,2]

Cardiac biomarker	No. of studies (no. of patients)	Sensitivity, % (95% CI)	Specificity, % (95% CI)	Diagnostic odds ratio (95% CI)
Initial presentation				
Troponin I*	4 (1149)	39 (10–78)	93 (88–97)	11 (3.4–34)
Troponin T	5 (1171)	44 (32–56)	92 (88–95)	9.5 (5.7–16)
CK-MB	10 (2504)	44 (35–53)	96 (94–97)	**
Serial evaluations				
Troponin I*	2 (1393)	90–100	83–96	230–460
Troponin T*	3 (904)	93 (85–97)	85 (76–91)	83 (33–210)
CK-MB	7 (3229)	80 (61–91)	96 (94–98)	**

CK-MB, creatinine kinase-MB.
* Includes all studies, not ED-specific studies; ** not reported.

more recent data. Also, cardiac biomarker assays have undergone refinements and advances that are not reflected in these studies. Two studies published by the New England Medical Center Evidence-based Practice Center provide summary data on the diagnostic performance/accuracy of cardiac biomarkers for studies performed in the ED setting with adult patients aged 18 years and older.[1,2] The report attempted to consolidate and interpret the explosion of publications since 1994, but also including relevant studies dating to 1966, that have attempted to evaluate various diagnostic technologies. Non-ED studies were included when there were no studies including ED patients. Table 18.1 shows the summary data for the diagnostic performances of CK-MB, troponin I, and troponin T. Data for ED-specific patients is shown separately when possible.

A single set of biomarkers obtained at ED presentation has poor sensitivity but high specificity for detecting AMI. Serial measurements greatly increase the sensitivity and maintain a high level of specificity. These data indicate that troponin I and troponin T, when compared to each other, have similar performance characteristics for the diagnosis of AMI, both at initial presentation and when assessed serially.

Another meta-analysis examined the predictive value of troponin I and troponin T for adverse events at 30 days, including death and AMI without ST-elevation in ACS.[3] The authors included published articles from Medline that included 30-day outcomes and serial biomarker assessments, and excluded patients who received thrombolytics. The authors present summary performances for each of the cardiac troponins, in addition to a comparison of performances for clinical trial and cohort studies. Seven studies including a total of 3579 patients were found that reported both troponin I and troponin T data. Two-hundred and sixty patients (7.2%) had an adverse event. The summary predictive sensitivity and specificity was 65% (95% CI: 58.9–70.8) and 74.5% (95% CI: 73–76), respectively, for troponin I, and 56.9% (95% CI: 50.7–63) and 76.9% (95% CI: 75.4–78.3), respectively, for troponin T. The summary negative predictive values, reflecting the prevalence of the outcomes, were 96.5% (95% CI: 95.7–97.1) for troponin I and 95.8% (95% CI: 95–96.5) for troponin T. There were no significant differences in the performance characteristics of either troponin biomarker when these studies were compared.

Heidenreich *et al.* examined the prognostic performance of troponin T and troponin I in clinical trials and cohort studies of patients with ACS.[4] A total of seven clinical trials and 19 cohort studies were found in their Medline search from 1966 to 1999. Studies that included only AMIs were excluded. The outcomes of death and death or AMI were reported. Two trials and two cohort studies compared troponin I and troponin T values directly, and the summary odds ratios for predicting mortality were similar [troponin I: OR 3.9 (95% CI: 2.3–6.6); troponin T: OR 5.2 (95% CI: 3.1–8.5)]. When troponin-positive death rates were compared between clinical trials and cohorts, using troponin I or troponin T, the cohort studies had higher summary odds ratios than the clinical trials, regardless of troponin subtype [troponin I: clinical trials summary OR 2.6 (95% CI: 1.8–3.6), cohort studies OR 8.5 (95% CI: 3.5–21.1), *P* <0.01; troponin T clinical trials summary OR 3.0 (95% CI: 1.6–5.5), cohort studies OR 5.1 (95% CI: 3.2–8.4), *P*<0.2].

Comments

Cardiac biomarkers are an integral part of the assessment for ACS in patients presenting with chest pain; however, they should not be the sole determinant. The studies we have reviewed showed poor sensitivity and high specificity for initial testing using the cardiac troponins, with serial testing leading to increased sensitivity. A positive result for troponin indicates higher short-term risks for the adverse outcomes of death and/or AMI. Results from cohort studies using either troponin I or troponin T show poorer short-term outcomes when compared to clinical trials, inferring that study-specific subject selection, patient heterogeneity, or trial conditions have an impact on the outcome.

Most EDs and hospital laboratories will run cardiac panels that typically include CK-MB and either troponin I or troponin T. Unless ST elevations, new left bundle branches, or dynamic ST segment changes are detected on the initial ECG, we advocate using cardiac troponin in the initial assessment of suspected ACS. A positive result for troponin should result in a cardiology evaluation, depending on the patient's medical history and presentation, and will often necessitate an evaluation of the coronary arteries, either invasively or non-invasively. Because of the biokinetic properties of the troponins, patients presenting acutely for the evaluation of chest pain may be negative for cardiac enzymes in the first instance. In these patients serial ECGs and serial cardiac biomarkers should be obtained. Among patients presenting with longer episodes of chest pain (hours to days) and with normal or non-diagnostic ECGs, the strategy of using a single troponin assessment in order to risk stratify them has not been adequately studied.

Non-invasive cardiac testing

There are several non-invasive tests that are commonly used in the assessment of CAD. Exercise ECG stress testing involves the assessment of a continuous ECG under an exercise protocol, often using a treadmill or bicycle. Dynamic ECG changes over time during the exercise process yield important and useful diagnostic information about the presence of underlying CAD. It is considered a low-cost test, is widely available, and can be performed and interpreted by a wide variety of non-cardiology physicians. Myocardial perfusion imaging with single-photon emission computed tomography (SPECT) uses a safe nuclear tracer (thallium-201 or technetium-99 sestamibi) that permits an evaluation of ventricular function, coronary artery perfusion, and regional blood flow. It is often coupled with a pharmacologic stressing agent that has vasodilatory effects—usually adenosine or dipyridamole—to enhance the diagnostic accuracy. Stress echocardiography in conjunction with either exercise alone or in combination with a pharmacological stressor, commonly dobutamine, permits the assessment of global cardiac and regional biventricular functions, transient regional wall motion abnormalities, and valvular dysfunction. Both SPECT imaging and echocardiography testing require specialized facilities for the preparation and execution of the study. Determining which one to use will be based on each individual patient, their exercise capacity, and study availability.

Clinical question two

"What are the performance characteristics for the following forms of non-invasive stress testing in diagnosing CAD: exercise ECG stress, stress echocardiography (exercise and pharmacologic), and stress myocardial perfusion imaging with SPECT?"

Numerous studies have examined the performances of the various non-invasive stress testing techniques. A meta-analysis of 147 studies of exercise EGC testing published from 1966 to 1987 was conducted by Gianrossi *et al.*[5] The exercise ECG was compared to coronary angiography for all 24 074 patients. The prevalence of CAD among the study patients was 66% based on the angiographic definition of having greater than 50% stenosis of a major coronary artery. There was wide variability in the performance characteristics across the studies. The summary sensitivity of the exercise ECG stress test was 68% ($\pm16\%$) and the summary specificity was 77% ($\pm17\%$) with a predictive accuracy of 73%. More recent data from another meta-analysis of exercise ECG stress information from 24 studies carried out between 1990 and 1997 with 2456 patients that had corresponding coronary angiography data, showed a summary sensitivity of 52% (95% CI: 50–55) and a summary specificity of 71% (95% CI: 68–74) for the detection of CAD.[6] The prevalence of CAD in this study was 69%.

Data extracted from several meta-analysis studies permit side-by-side comparisons of exercise and vasodilator echocardiography studies (Table 18.2). The data show a higher sensitivity of stress echocardiography when used with SPECT imaging, whereas the use of vasodilators (adenosine or dipyridamole) maximizes specificity for diagnosing CAD.

Kim *et al.* compared the different pharmacologic agents used in combination with either echocardiography or SPECT stress testing in a meta-analysis for the diagnosis of CAD (Table 18.3).[8] Patients had to have undergone either type of stress test and coronary angiography. Studies that included patients imaged following known AMI, post-angioplasty, or post-coronary artery bypass grafting were excluded. Dobutamine was most commonly used in

Table 18.2 Summary performance characteristics of stress echocardiography results from meta-analyses

	Ref.	No. patients	No. studies	CAD prevalence (%)	Sensitivity, % (95% CI)	Specificity, % (95% CI)
Exercise	7	533	8	74	79	82
stress echo	6	2637	24	66	85 (83–87)	77 (74–80)
Dipyridamole	7	533	8	74	72	92
stress echo	8	1835	20	67	70 (66–74)	93 (90–95)
Adenosine stress echo	8	516	6	73	72 (62–79)	91 (88–93)

CAD, coronary artery disease.

Table 18.3 Summary performance test characteristics of different pharmacologic agents coupled with echocardiography or single-photon emission computed tomography (SPECT) stress testing in published studies, 1975–1999, from Kim et al. 2001[8]

	No. studies (no. patients)	CAD prevalence, %	Sensitivity, % (95% CI)	Specificity, % (95% CI)
Echocardiography stress				
Adenosine	6 (516)	73	72 (62–79)	91 (88–93)
Dipyridamole	20 (1835)	67	70 (66–74)	93 (90–95)
Dobutamine	40 (4097)	70	80 (77–83)	84 (80–86)
SPECT stress				
Adenosine	9 (1207)	80	90 (89–92)	75 (70–79)
Dipyridamole	21 (1464)	71	89 (84–93)	65 (54–74)
Dobutamine	14 (1066)	66	82 (77–87)	75 (70–79)

CAD, coronary artery disease.

combination with echocardiography and had a higher sensitivity but lower specificity when compared to adenosine and dipyridamole studies. Conversely, dipyridamole was most commonly used together with SPECT imaging with higher sensitivity but also lower specificity compared to dobutamine.

Women have been under-represented in the majority of non-invasive stress testing studies throughout the 20th century. Because the majority of studies examined middle-aged men who have an overall higher prevalence of CAD, there have been concerns about the application of the various stress test modalities to women. Fortunately, once CAD is recognized, treatments and interventions are similar for both sexes; but for the clinician the concern about gender bias in the literature is a reasonable one.

Kwok et al. examined studies published from 1966 to 1995 that included at least 50 women who underwent a minimum of one type of exercise stress test and who had corresponding coronary angiography information.[9] Studies that did not present female-specific data were not included, nor were non-English studies or studies done for post-myocardial infarction or post-angioplasty evaluations. A total of 21 studies involving 4113 patients were included in the meta-analysis with a mean CAD prevalence of 39% (see Table 18.4). These data demonstrated that none of the non-invasive exercise stress tests were highly sensitive or specific in women. Stress echocardiography demonstrated the highest sensitivity and specificity but was also the least studied modality in this report.

Dutch researchers examined the dobutamine stress echocardiography among women in a meta-analysis of 14 studies between 1992 and 2002 in which there was corresponding coronary angiography data.[10] In six of the

Table 18.4 Summary performance characteristics of the various exercise stress tests among women from Kwok et al. 1999[9]

	No. studies (no. patients)	Sensitivity, % (95% CI)	Specificity, % (95% CI)	LR+ ratio, % (95% CI)	LR– ratio, % (95% CI)
ECG	19 (3721)	61 (54–68)	70 (64–75)	2.3 (1.8–2.7)	0.6 (0.5–0.6)
Radionuclide (thallium)	5 (842)	78 (72–83)	64 (51–77)	2.9 (1.0–5.0)	0.4 (0.3–0.4)
Echocardiography	3 (296)	86 (75–96)	79 (72–86)	4.3 (2.9–5.7)	0.2 (0.1–0.3)

ECG, electrocardiogram; LR, likelihood ratio.

Table 18.5 Summary weighted test characteristics of stress tests from Geleijnse et al. 2007[10]

	No. studies (no. patients)	CAD prevalence, %	Sensitivity %*	Specificity %*
All dobutamine stress echo	14 (901)	48	72	88
Studies comparing dobutamine stress echo by sex				
Females	7 (482)	59	77	81
Males	7 (966)	73	77	77
Studies comparing dobutamine stress echo to stress nuclear scintigraphy				
Echocardiography	6 (379)	**	77	90
Nuclear	6 (372)	**	73	70

CAD, coronary artery disease.
* 95% confidence intervals not provided; ** data not provided.

studies, direct comparisons between male and female subjects could be made. The researchers were also able to compare dobutamine stress echocardiography to stress nuclear scintigraphy in six studies. The results from the meta-analysis are shown in Table 18.5. The performance of dobutamine stress echocardiography was similar among men and women in the studies reviewed. Interestingly, dobutamine stress echo had substantially higher specificity in women compared to stress nuclear scintigraphy. It has been postulated that breast tissue attenuation artifact, a smaller ventricle size in women, and estrogen-related effects on endothelial tissues all may contribute to the false positive tests in women (and hence the lower specificity).

Comments

Non-invasive stress testing is currently recommended in patients that are suspected of having CAD but are not currently exhibiting any ECG or enzymatic evidence of AMI or UA. Exercise ECG is the most widely available form of stress testing but suffers from a lack of sufficiently high sensitivity or specificity. However, in cases when clinicians have a low to very low suspicion of CAD, it is a reasonable first step stress test. If the facilities and resources for exercise imaging or other imaging modes are available, additional information can be obtained with better test performances. Pharmacologic additions to the stress tests enhance diagnostic accuracy and can be used in those patients incapable of exercising. Vasodilator drugs such as adenosine and dipyridamole can maximize sensitivity when combined with SPECT imaging, whereas when combined with echocardiography the specificity is maximized. For women, stress echocardiography with dobutamine appears to have better specificity compared to stress nuclear scintigraphy methods.

CT coronary angiography

CT angiography of the coronary vessels for the purposes of identifying potential ACS is among the most recently developed diagnostic modality to assess patients with chest pain in the ED. Advances in CT technology with improved spatial and temporal resolution have permitted the acquisition of detailed pictures of the coronary anatomy to detect coronary artery stenosis as well as calcified and non-calcified coronary artery plaques.

Clinical question three

"How do the test characteristics of multi-detector CT (MDCT) angiography compare with conventional invasive coronary angiography?"
Three meta-analyses, all published in 2006, have examined this question and have come to the same general conclusion. The first study by Dutch researchers examined original studies published between 2000 and 2005 in which at least 20 patients with native coronary arteries were involved, and in which both MDCT and coronary angiography were performed.[11] Fifteen studies were found, totaling 944 patients. The mean prevalence of CAD in the studies was 59% (range 31–81%). The pooled patient-based sensitivity for the 10 studies reporting patient-based data was 89% (95% CI: 85–92). The pooled negative likelihood ratio was 0.16 (95% CI: 0.10–0.26).

Another study by European researchers evaluated studies from 2002 to 2006 that reported results with at least 30 patients that had undergone both MDCT and coronary angiography studies.[12] The MDCTs had to employ the newer generation CT technology (≥16 slices). A total of 27 studies were included in the analysis, permitting analysis at the coronary segment, vessel, and patient levels. The results are summarized in Table 18.6.

Table 18.6 Pooled performance characteristics of multi-detector computed tomography angiography compared to coronary angiography, based on the meta-analysis from Hamon *et al.* 2006[12]

	Level of analysis		
	Coronary segment (n = 22 789)	Coronary vessel (n = 2726)	Patient (n = 1570)
Sensitivity, % (95% CI)	81 (72–89)	82 (80–85)	96 (94–98)
Specificity, % (95% CI)	93 (90–97)	91 (90–92)	74 (65–84)
LR+ (95% CI)	22 (13–35)	12 (7–21)	5 (3–8)
LR– (95% CI)	0.11 (0.06–0.21)	0.08 (0.02–0.32)	0.05 (0.03–0.09)

LR, likelihood ratio.

Table 18.7 Pooled performance characteristics of multi-detector computed tomography angiography compared to coronary angiography, based on the meta-analysis from Sun and Jiang 2006[13]

	Level of analysis		
	Coronary segment (n = 34 studies)	Coronary vessel (n = 16 studies)	Patient (n = 21 studies)
Sensitivity, % (95% CI)	83 (79–89)	90 (87–94)	91 (88–95)
Specificity, % (95% CI)	93 (91–96)	87 (80–93)	86 (81–92)

The largest meta-analysis comes from Sun and Jiang who examined 47 studies from 1998 to 2006.[13] The studies included reports with 10 or more patients who underwent MDCT and coronary angiography. The studies included used CTs with between 4 and 64 detectors. Table 18.7 summarizes the results; the prevalence of CAD was found to be 74% (95% CI: 64–84).

Comments

The three published meta-analyses on the topic of the diagnostic performance of MDCT angiography consistently show that the sensitivity is in the mid 80–90% range, and increases as one moves from the coronary segment level to the patient level. Conversely, the specificity is in the mid 80–90% range and decreases as one moves from the coronary segment to the patient level. An important element to keep in mind when interpreting this data is that almost none of the studies included in the meta-analyses examined ED patients presenting acutely for evaluation of chest pain.

A review by Hollander and Litt of the six small cohort studies to date that have examined the use of CT coronary angiography in the evaluation of ED patients considered low risk for ACS, indicate that non-invasive CT coronary angiography is at least as sensitive and specific as stress myocardial perfusion imaging for the exclusion or detection of ACS, and that it has the potential to decrease the overall time required to complete an evaluation, and has no short-term adverse outcomes associated with its use or with missed diagnoses.[14] The major limitation of the reviewed studies is the small sample sizes (the number of enrolled patients ranged from 40 to 197). This modality has the potential to significantly speed up the evaluation process and is a research area that holds promise in the evaluation of low-risk ACS patients.

References

1. Lau, J., Ioannidis, J.P.A., Balk, E.M., *et al.* (2001) Diagnosing acute cardiac ischemia in the emergency department: a systematic review of the accuracy and clinical effect of current technology. *Annals of Emergency Medicine* **37**(5): 453–460.
2. Balk, E.M., Ioannidis, J.P.A., Salem, D., Chew, P.W. and Lau, J. (2001) Accuracy of biomarkers to diagnose acute cardiac ischemia in the emergency department: a meta-analysis. *Annals of Emergency Medicine* **37**(5): 478–494.
3. Fleming, S.M. and Daly, K.M. (2001) Cardiac troponins in suspected acute coronary syndrome. *Cardiology* **95**: 66–73.
4. Heidenreich, P.A., Alloggiamento, T., Melsop, K., McDonald, K.M., Go, A.S. and Hlatky, M.A. (2001) The prognostic value of troponin in patients with non-ST elevation acute coronary syndromes: a meta-analysis. *Journal of American College of Cardiology* **38**(2): 478–485.
5. Gianrossi, R., Detrano, R., Muvihill, D., *et al.* (1989) Exercise-induced ST depression in the diagnosis of coronary artery disease. *Circulation* **80**(1): 87–98.
6. Fleischmann, K.E., Hunink, M.G., Kuntz, K.M. and Douglas, P.S. (1998) Exercise echocardiography or exercise SPECT imaging? A meta-analysis of diagnostic test performance. *Journal of the American Medical Association* **280**(10): 913–920.
7. Fonseca, L.A. and Picano, E. (2001) Comparison of dipyridamole and exercise stress echocardiography for detection of coronary artery disease (a meta-analysis). *American Journal of Cardiology* **87**: 1193–1196.
8. Kim, C., Kwok, Y.S., Heagerty, P. and Redberg, R. (2001) Pharmacologic stress testing for coronary artery disease diagnosis: a meta-analysis. *American Heart Journal* **142**(6): 934–944.
9. Kwok, Y., Kim, C., Grady, D., Segal, M. and Redberg, R. (1999) Meta-analysis of exercise testing to detect coronary artery disease in women. *American Journal of Cardiology* **83**: 660–666.
10. Geleijnse, M.L., Krenning, B.J., Soliman, O., II, Nemes, A., Galema, T.W. and ten Cate, F.J. (2007) Dobutamine stress echocardiography for the detection of coronary artery disease in women. *American Journal of Cardiology* **99**: 714–717.

11. van der Zaag-Loonen, H.J., Dikkers, R., de Bock, G.H. and Oudkerk, M. (2006) The clinical value of a negative multi-detector computed tomographic angiography in patients suspected of coronary artery disease: a meta-analysis. *European Radiology* **16**: 2748–2756.

12. Hamon, M., Biondi-Zoccai, G.G.L., Malagutti, P., *et al.* (2006) Diagnostic performance of multislice spiral computed tomography of coronary arteries as compared with conventional invasive coronary angiography. *Journal of American College of Cardiology* **48**(9): 1896–1910.

13. Sun, Z. and Jiang, W. (2006) Diagnostic value of multislice computed tomography angiography in coronary artery disease: a meta-analysis. *European Journal of Radiology* **60**: 279–286.

14. Hollander, J.E. and Litt, H.I. (2006) Computerized tomographic coronary angiography for the evaluation of ED patients with potential acute coronary syndromes. *Emergency Medicine Cardiac Research and Education Group International.* Available at: http://www.emcreg.org/education/cme/cme.html

SECTION 4
Infectious Disease

Chapter 19 **Serious Bacterial Infections and Occult Bacteremia in Children**

Highlights

- The principle goal of the emergency department (ED) evaluation of the febrile infant under three years of age is to identify patients at risk for serious bacterial infection (SBI) and occult bacteremia.
- Two clinical decision rules, the Philadelphia protocol and Rochester criteria, are sensitive rules for identifying febrile infants at low risk from SBI.
- Successful vaccination programs against *Haemophilus influenzae* type B (HIB) and *Streptococcus pneumoniae* have resulted in lower rates of occult bacteremia in febrile infants.

Background

About 20% of febrile children (under 3 years old) will have no source of infection after a thorough physical examination. A small percentage of febrile children will have an SBI, which encompasses bacteremia, bacterial gastroenteritis, cellulitis, meningitis, osteomyelitis, pneumonia, septic arthritis, and urinary tract infection. The challenge in the ED is to identify children with fevers who are at risk of SBI and who need more testing, empirical antibiotics, and/or inpatient admission for observation. Several large studies have examined various criteria to differentiate the risk of SBI for children with fever.

In general, children who are 0–28 days old have a high prevalence of a serious occult source of infection and should receive a full sepsis work-up (including laboratory screening, urinalysis, and lumbar puncture) and empirical antibiotics. For children who are between 29 and 60 days old there are clinical decision rules to identify children who are at low risk (the Philadelphia

Evidence-Based Emergency Care: Diagnostic Testing and Clinical Decision Rules. By J.M. Pines and W.W. Everett. Published 2008 by Blackwell Publishing, ISBN: 978-14051-5400-0.

protocol and Rochester criteria). For children who are not low risk, the recommendations are to hospitalize them, do a full work-up, and empirically treat. For those deemed to be low risk, discharging them on the condition that they can receive a close follow-up is recommended. Between two and three months old there is a grey zone with differing approaches used, ranging from urinalysis testing to empirical treatment with intramuscular antibiotics.

Children between the ages of 3 and 36 months that have no focal source of infection are at risk of occult bacteremia. This is defined as the presence of bacteria in the blood in a febrile child that otherwise appears to be well and that has no focus of infection, and is a source of controversy in the ED. Occult bactermia is more frequent in children with high white blood cell (WBC) counts (>15 000/mm^3) and elevated temperatures (>39°C). Therefore, for a child that appears toxic, has a high fever, and an elevated WBC count >15, bandemia, or a high absolute neutrophil count (ANC), a full work-up (including a lumbar puncture where meningitis is a concern) should be performed, antibiotics prescribed and the child admitted. However, non-toxic children who do not have elevated ANCs may be considered as candidates for outpatient management.

The advent of two vaccines against HIB and *Streptococcus pneumoniae* has changed the epidemiology of occult bacteremia. In the pre-HIB era, the prevalence ranged from about 3 to 12%. The most frequent cause was *Streptococcus pneumoniae* (60–85%), while HIB was responsible for approximately 5–20%. A recent study has estimated the prevalence of occult bacteremia to be less than 2%.

Clinical question one

"What are the Philadelphia protocol and the Rochester criteria and how do these clinical decision rules differentiate children less than two months old with SBI?"
The derivation of the Philadelphia protocol involved a study of 747 consecutive infants who were between 29 and 56 days old and that had temperatures of 38.2°C or above.[1] A total of 460 infants had laboratory or clinical findings indicating SBI and were hospitalized and treated empirically with antibiotics. The authors used the following screening criteria for SBI: a WBC count in excess of 15 000/mm^3; a spun urine specimen with more than 10 WBC per high-power field or that was positive under bright-field microscopy; a cerebrospinal fluid (CSF) with a WBC count greater than 8/mm^3 or a positive Gram's stain; or an infiltrate on chest radiography. The 287 infants with normal physical examinations and normal laboratory findings were assigned to either inpatient observation without antibiotics, or outpatient care with a close follow-up. A total of 65 infants (9%) had SBI and 64 were identified

using the screening criteria. The sensitivity was 98% (95% CI: 92–100). Of the 287 who were low risk, only one had SBI. The authors termed these criteria the Philadelphia protocol, which states that children are low risk if all of the following are met:

- a WBC count below 15 000 with a band cell count of less than 20%;
- a WBC count of less than 10 per high-power field in urinalysis;
- a WBC count for the CSF of less than 7/mm^3; and
- a negative chest radiography.

More recently the same authors performed a three-year prospective cohort study of the Philadelphia protocol.[2] They followed 422 infants who were between 29 and 60 days old and had a fever exceeding 38°C. A total of 101 infants (24%) were identified as low risk and safe for outpatient management. The authors reported that of the 43 children with SBI, none were identified as low risk by the Philadelphia protocol.

The initial derivation of the Rochester criteria involved a two-year study of 233 infants aged three months or younger.[3] Term infants with no perinatal complications or serious underlying diseases, or who had previously received antibiotics were included. A total of 144 (62%) were considered unlikely to have an SBI, in that they did not have any physical examination findings consistent with ear, soft tissue or skeletal infections, and had a WBC count of 5000–15 000/mm^3, less than 1500 band cells/mm^3, and a normal urinalysis. Of the 144, only one infant had an SBI (0.7%) compared to 22 (25%) in the high-risk group. No patients in the low-risk group had bacteremia compared with 9% in the high-risk group. They termed these criteria the Rochester criteria and stated that there is a low risk if the infant:

- was full-term;
- was previously healthy;
- has a WBC count of 5000–15 000/mm^3 with less than 1500 band cells/mm^3; and
- has a WBC count of less than 10 per high-power field in urinalysis.

The same authors then prospectively examined the criteria in a study a few years later (1988).[4] They enrolled 237 previously healthy infants aged three months or younger with fever. A total of 149 (63%) were low risk by the following criteria: no findings of soft tissue or skeletal infections, no otitis media, normal urinalysis, less than 25 WBC per high-power field on stool examination, and a WBC count of 5000–15 000/mm^3 with less than 1500 band cells/mm^3. None of the low-risk patients had SBI compared with 24% of the high-risk patients, and 8% had bacteremia.

A reappraisal of the Philadelphia protocol and the Rochester criteria was recently published.[5] The study involved infants aged 56 days or younger with a rectal temperature of greater than 38.1°C. As part of the study protocol the physicians gave their overall impression of sepsis and scored each infant using an Infant Observation Score. They assigned 188 infants to the Philadelphia protocol and 259 to the Rochester criteria. The negative predictive value of the Philadelphia protocol was 97.1% (95 CI: 85.1–99.8) and that of the Rochester criteria was 97.3% (95% CI: 90.5–99.2). The authors concluded that the Philadelphia protocol and the Rochester criteria both had high negative predictive values, similar to the initial derivation and validation studies.

Clinical question two

"How well does the Philadelphia protocol work when applied to children of less than 29 days of age?"
The Philadelphia protocol was applied retrospectively to a cohort of 254 infants younger than 29 days who were admitted for evaluation of SBI.[6] The overall prevalence of SBI was 12.6%. A total of 109 (43%) of infants could have been classified as low risk by the Philadelphia protocol. Five children were found to have an SBI that would have been missed by the Philadelphia protocol. The authors warned that these results demonstrate the unpredictable nature of SBI in infants less than 29 days of age.

Clinical question three

"What is the utility of laboratory testing to discriminate children with occult bacteremia?"
In 1998, Kuppermann *et al.* studied a large cohort of 6579 outpatients aged 3–36 months with temperatures of 39°C and higher in 10 US hospitals between 1987 and 1991 to examine predictors for occult pneumococcal bacteremia.[7] A total of 164 patients (2.5%) had occult pneumococcal bacteremia (OPB). The authors performed a split derivation and validation to derive a model for predicting the presence of OPB. In univariable analysis, they reported that patients with occult bacteremia were younger, more frequently ill-appearing, and had higher temperatures, WBC counts, ANCs, and absolute band cell counts than patients without bacteremia. In the multivariable analysis three variables were independently significant: (i) ANC with an odds ration (OR) of 1.15 (95% CI: 1.06–1.25) for each increase of 1000 cells/mm^3; (ii) temperature with an OR of 1.77 (95% CI: 1.21–2.58) for each 1°C increase; and (iii) age younger than two years with an OR of 2.43 (95% CI: 1.11–5.3). They reported that 8.1% of patients with an ANC greater than 10 000 cells/mm^3 had occult bacteremia compared to 0.8% of those with a count less than 10 000 cells/mm^3.

Clinical question four

"In the age of pneumococcal conjugate vaccination are vaccinated children still at risk of pneumoccocal bacteremia?"
A recent study sought to answer this question. The authors performed a non-concurrent prospective observational cohort study.[8] They enrolled patients aged less than 36 months with temperatures exceeding 38°C. Of 3571 eligible patients, 1428 had blood cultures. Of those, 833 had received at least one immunization with a heptavalent pneumococcal vaccine. In the group that had received the vaccine, no patients had positive pneumococcal blood cultures compared with 13 (2.4%) in the non-immunized group.

Comment

The majority of children who are evaluated for fever when aged three years or younger will have a self-limited viral illness. Before the advent of the HIB and pneumococcal conjugate vaccines about 10% of these children with an unknown source of infection had occult bacteremia and SBI. Recent studies have found lower rates of SBI (<2%). It appears clear, though, that any infant who is younger than 29 days old should have a full work-up, and be admitted and treated with empirical antibiotics. Children who appear non-toxic, between 1 and 36 months old, with no apparent source of fever, and who have received their vaccinations, can undergo risk stratification through laboratory analysis and can be sent home with close follow-up. However, many of the studies that used the Philadelphia protocol and Rochester criteria are small single-center studies and have not been validated in large cohorts of children.

In light of recent change in the microbiology of infection in this age group because of the reduced rates of infection by pneumoccous and HIB, evaluation and treatment recommendations are certainly evolving and may be modified as newer data is published. However, we recommend a cautious approach to every febrile child under three years old because of the potential for poor outcomes in the case of untreated SBI.

References

1. Baker, M.D., Bell, L.M. and Avner, J.R. (1993) Outpatient management without antibiotics of fever in selected infants. *New England Journal of Medicine* **329**(20): 1437–1441.
2. Baker, M.D., Bell, L.M. and Avner, J.R. (1999) The efficacy of routine outpatient management without antibiotics of fever in selected infants. *Pediatrics* **103**(3): 627–631.

3. Dagan, R., Powell, K.R., Hall, C.B. and Menegus, M.A. (1985) Identification of infants unlikely to have serious bacterial infection although hospitalized for suspected sepsis. *Journal of Pediatrics* **107**(6): 855–860.
4. Dagan, R., Sofer, S., Phillip, M. and Shachak, E. (1988) Ambulatory care of febrile infants younger than 2 months of age classified as being at low risk for having serious bacterial infections. *Journal of Pediatrics* **112**(3): 355–360.
5. Garra, G., Cunningham, S.J. and Crain, E.F. (2005) Reappraisal of criteria used to predict serious bacterial illness in febrile infants less than 8 weeks of age. *Academic Emergency Medicine* **12**(10): 921–925.
6. Baker, M.D. and Bell, L.M. (1999) Unpredictability of serious bacterial infections in febrile infants from birth to 1 month of age. *Archives of Pediatric Adolescent Medicine* **153**: 508–511.
7. Kuppermann, N., Fleisher, G.R. and Jaffe, D.M. (1998) Predictors of occult pneumococcal bacteremia in young febrile children. *Annals of Emergency Medicine* **31**: 679–687.
8. Carstairs, K.L., Tanen, D.A., Johnson, A.S., Kailes, S.B. and Riffenburgh, R.H. (2007) Pneumococcal bacteremia in febrile infants presenting to the emergency department before and after the introduction of the heptavalent pneumococcal vaccine. *Annals of Emergency Medicine* **49**(6): 772–777.

Chapter 20 **Bacterial Meningitis in Children**

Highlights

- All children suspected of having meningitis should undergo a lumbar puncture.
- The Bacterial Meningitis Score (BMS) is a simple decision rule that discriminates bacterial meningitis from aseptic meningitis with high sensitivity in children with cerebrospinal fluid (CSF) pleocytosis.

Background

Meningitis in a child can be suspected based upon history and physical examination alone, but confirming the diagnosis requires a lumbar puncture and examination of the CSF. CSF pleocytosis is defined as a CSF white blood cell (WBC) count of 10 cells/μL or above, with a correction made for the presence of CSF red blood cells (RBCs) using a 1:500 ratio of leukocytes to erythrocytes. When evaluating a child with CSF pleocytosis, the most common diagnosis is aseptic meningitis (in more than 80–90% of cases); however, bacterial meningitis is still present in a small proportion of patients. Completely excluding bacterial meningitis requires a negative CSF culture (which takes 2–3 days). When there is CSF pleocytosis, most children are admitted for broad spectrum antibiotics while waiting for culture results. The advent of two vaccines, the *Haemophilus influenzae* type B (HIB) and the pneumoccoal conjugate vaccines, have significantly reduced the incidence of bacterial meningitis in children in the US. Because the prevalence of bacterial meningitis in children with CSF pleocytosis is low, a clinical decision rule to identify children that are at very low risk for meningitis at the time of clinical presentation may limit unnecessary hospital admissions and antibiotic use in aseptic meningitis.

Evidence-Based Emergency Care: Diagnostic Testing and Clinical Decision Rules. By J.M. Pines and W.W. Everett. Published 2008 by Blackwell Publishing, ISBN: 978-14051-5400-0.

The BMS was recently validated across 20 academic medical centers in the post-HIB and post-pneuococcal vaccine era. While there have been many other clinical decision rules derived to answer this question, most have not been internally or externally validated. In addition, many rules were published in the pre-HIB and pre-pneumococcal vaccine eras.

Clinical question

"What is the BMS and how can this be used to rule out bacterial meningitis at the time of clinical presentation in children with CSF pleocytosis?"

The BMS was developed by Nigrovic and colleagues to classify patients with CSF pleocytosis who are at very low risk of bacterial meningitis.[1] This clinical decision rule states that patients are at very low risk of bacterial meningitis if they lack all of the following criteria:

- a positive CSF Gram stain;
- a CSF absolute neutrophil count (ANC) of 1000 cells/μL or above;
- a CSF protein level of 80 mg/dL or above;
- a peripheral blood ANC of 10 000 cells/μL or above; and
- a history of seizure before or at the time of presentation.

The BMS was derived from a study of 696 children aged from 29 days to 19 years old who were hospitalized with CSF pleocytosis at one center. The overall prevalence of bacterial meningitis was 18%. The authors performed a split derivation and validation study and used multivariable logistic regression and recursive partitioning to derive the clinical prediction rule. A BMS was calculated by giving two points for a positive CSF Gram stain and one point for each other variables, if present. They found that a BMS equal to zero identified patients with aseptic meningitis with 100% accuracy and did not misclassify any child with bacterial meningitis in the validation set. The negative predictive value for a score of zero was 100% (95% CI: 97–100) and a BMS of two or above predicted the presence of bacterial meningitis with a sensitivity of 87% (95% CI: 72–96).

The BMS was recently validated using a multicenter retrospective cohort study in 20 US academic medical centers.[2] This included all children between the ages of 29 days and 19 years old who presented from January 2001 to June 2004 with CSF pleocytosis, and who had not received any antibiotics prior to lumbar puncture. In 3295 patients with CSF pleocytosis, 3.7% (95% CI: 3.1–4.4) had bacterial meningitis and the remainder had aseptic meningitis. There were 1714 children who were categorized as low risk by the BMS (i.e. score = 0). Of those, two were identified with bacterial meningitis at a sensitivity of 98.3% (95% CI: 94.2–99.8) and a negative predictive value of 99.9% (95% CI: 99.6–100). Both of the patients with bacterial meningitis and BMS scores of zero were less than two months old. From this, the authors concluded that the BMS is an accurate clinical decision rule that imparts a very low risk of bacterial meningitis (0.1%) in patients with none of the criteria listed above.

Comment

In a large multicenter study, the BMS seemed to accurately discriminate children with CSF pleocytosis and aseptic meningitis from those with bacterial meningitis, with close to 100% sensitivity. The BMS is a simple and easy to use scoring system that involves routinely collected data. This may be very helpful to clinicians in distinguishing children with pleocytosis that may be candidates for outpatient management because they have a very low likelihood of bacterial meningitis. There has been an external validation of the BMS in two small studies in France which confirmed a sensitivity of almost 100%.[3]

There are two considerations that must be taken into account when using the BMS to guide clinical management. First, because the BMS was designed to identify patients at low risk for bacterial meningitis only, some patients who may benefit from antimicrobial therapy, such as those with Lyme meningitis and herpes simplex virus encephalitis may not be captured by the BMS. We therefore recommend that the BMS be used in conjunction with a clinical assessment of the patient for other important and treatable infections. Second, because the two cases of meningitis that were missed by the BMS in the multicenter validation study involved children under two months of age, we would recommend exercising caution when applying the BMS to this high-risk population.

References

1. Nigrovic, L.E., Kuppermann, N. and Malley, R. (2002) Development and validation of a multivariable predictive model to distinguish bacterial from aseptic meningitis in children in the post-*Haemophilus influenzae* era. *Pediatrics* **110**: 712–719.
2. Nigrovic, L.E., Kuppermann, N., Macias, C.G., *et al.* (2007) Clinical prediction rule for identifying children with cerebrospinal fluid pleocytosis at very low risk of bacterial meningitis. *Journal of the American Medical Association* **297**: 52–60.
3. Dubos, F., Lamotte, B., Bibi-Triki, F., *et al.* (2006) Clinical decision rules to distinguish between bacterial and aseptic meningitis. *Archives of Disease in Childhood* **91**: 647–650.

Chapter 21 **Necrotizing Fasciitis**

Highlights

- Necrotizing fasciitis is a rare but potentially lethal condition that requires early recognition and aggressive surgical treatment.
- The Laboratory Risk Indicator for Necrotizing Fasciitis (LRINEC) score uses routine blood test results that can discriminate necrotizing fasciitis from severe cellulitis/abscess.
- The LRINEC criteria still need to be validated in an external setting before widespread use can be recommended.

Background

Necrotizing fasciitis is a rapidly progressive infection involving the fascia and subcutaneous tissue (Fig. 21.1). Differentiating necrotizing fasciitis from other skin and soft tissue infections is important in the emergency department (ED) because while necrotizing fasciitis is a rare disease, it can result in high morbidity and mortality rates. According to some reports, mortality as a result of necrotizing fasciitis can approach 34%. Necrotizing fasciitis is a surgical disease and the early recognition and debridement of necrotic fascia and other involved areas are major determinants of overall outcome (Fig. 21.2). A delay in debridement has been associated with poorer survival.

Early on, necrotizing fasciitis can be difficult to distinguish from other forms of soft tissue infections, such as cellulitis and abscess. While computed tomography, magnetic resonance imaging, and ultrasound have been shown to be useful in distinguishing necrotizing fasciitis from other clinical entities, the choice of which patients to perform either rule-out or rule-in imaging studies on has been a source of controversy.

Evidence-Based Emergency Care: Diagnostic Testing and Clinical Decision Rules. By J.M. Pines and W.W. Everett. Published 2008 by Blackwell Publishing, ISBN: 978-14051-5400-0.

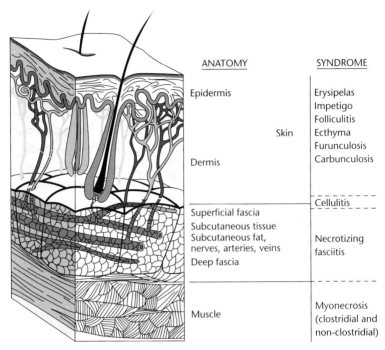

ANATOMY		SYNDROME
Epidermis		Erysipelas
		Impetigo
		Folliculitis
	Skin	Ecthyma
		Furunculosis
Dermis		Carbunculosis
		Cellulitis
Superficial fascia		
Subcutaneous tissue		
Subcutaneous fat, nerves, arteries, veins		Necrotizing fasciitis
Deep fascia		
Muscle		Myonecrosis (clostridial and non-clostridial)

Figure 21.1 Schematic of the different layers of skin and the corresponding infections associated with each layer.

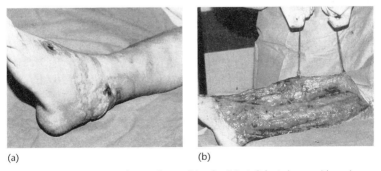

(a)   (b)

Figure 21.2 (a) A suspected case of necrotizing fasciitis. Left foot shown with oozing wound, dusky skin, and bullae formation. (b) Surgical exploration resulted in extensive debridement. (Source: Hall *et al. Principles of Critical Care* 3rd Edition © 2005. Reproduced with permission of The McGraw-Hill Companies.)

Clinical question

"What are the LRINEC criteria and how can they be used in the ED to distinguish necrotizing fasciitis from other skin and soft tissue infections?"

The LRINEC investigators developed a scoring system to differentiate necrotizing fasciitis from other skin and soft tissue infections.[1] They performed a retrospective study in two teaching hospitals in Singapore using a cohort of 314 patients to derive the LRINEC scoring system, and a cohort of 140 patients to validate it. They included 140 patients who had necrotizing fasciitis and 309 patients with severe cellulitis or abscesses. They found that white blood cell counts, hemoglobin, sodium, glucose, creatinine, and C-reactive protein levels were associated with a diagnosis of necrotizing fasciitis. The authors constructed the LRINEC score through conversion of the independent predictors of necrotizing fasciitis into an integer scoring system, which is detailed in Table 21.1.

Using a cutoff of six points or higher, there was a positive predictive value of 92% and a negative predictive value of 96%. The area under the receiver operator curve was 0.98 in the derivation set and 0.976 in the validation cohort, showing a high degree of accuracy in differentiating necrotizing fasciitis from cellulitis/abscess.

Comment

The LRINEC score demonstrated good discrimination in the clinical detection of early cases of necrotizing fasciitis in the derivation and validation cohorts from two academic medical centers in Singapore. The LRINEC has

Table 21.1 The Laboratory Risk Indicator for Necrotizing Fasciitis (LRINEC) score to differentiate necrotizing fasciitis from severe cellulitis from Wong *et al.*[1]

Variable	Value	Score*
C-reactive protein (mg/L)	≥150	4
WBC (mm^{-3})	15–25	1
WBC (mm^{-3})	>25	2
Hemoglobin	11–13.5	1
Hemoglobin	<11	2
Sodium (mmol/L)	<135	2
Creatinine (mg/dL)	>1.6	2
Glucose (mg/dL)	>180	1

WBC, white blood cell.
* A score >6 is regarded as being a positive test.

not yet been validated in a separate population; however, given its high accuracy in differentiating necrotizing fasciitis from other less severe infections, ED physicians should consider using the LRINEC scoring system or the laboratory abnormalities detailed within it, along with their clinical evaluation, in selecting patients for imaging studies to rule out necrotizing fasciitis.

Reference

1. Wong, C.H., Khin, L.W., Heng, K.S., *et al.* (2004) The LRINEC (Laboratory Risk Indicator for Necrotizing Fasciitis) score: a tool for distinguishing necrotizing fasciitis from other soft tissue infections based on routine laboratory testing. *Critical Care Medical* **32**(7): 1535–1541.

Chapter 22 **Pharyngitis**

Highlights

- Differentiating bacterial pharyngitis (group A streptococci; GAS) from other causes of sore throat is a clinical challenge.
- The Centor criteria can predict the probability of a GAS infection based on clinical criteria.
- Patients with intermediate scores may benefit from confirmatory rapid strep testing or cultures before starting therapy, to avoid the overtreatment of viral infections.

Background

The complaint of sore throat is common in emergency medicine. The most common bacterial cause for sore throat is GAS. The prevalence of GAS pharyngitis in patients with sore throat is 15–36% for children and 5–17% for adults. The value of using antibiotics has been debated in this disease because it usually resolves spontaneously, without complications. However, antibiotics are recommended in cases where there is a high likelihood of, or culture-confirmed, streptococcal infection of the throat.

The reasons for treating patients with antibiotics are to prevent complications, reduce symptoms, and to prevent the transmission of disease to others. A recent Cochrane review found that at three days antibiotics reduced symptoms of sore throat, headache and fever.[1] Complications following GAS pharyngitis include suppurative (acute otitis media and sinusitis) and non-suppurative (acute glomerulonephritis and rheumatic fever) complications. In general, antibiotics tend to reduce the incidence of suppurative complications considerably—by about a quarter in acute otitis media and by about a

Evidence-Based Emergency Care: Diagnostic Testing and Clinical Decision Rules. By J.M. Pines and W.W. Everett. Published 2008 by Blackwell Publishing, ISBN: 978-14051-5400-0.

half in acute sinusitis. Antibiotics reduce the likelihood of rheumatic fever by about a third.

There are no standardized diagnostic testing guidelines to follow when deciding which emergency department (ED) patients with a sore throat require antibiotic therapy. However, many of the guidelines available base their strategy on a clinical scoring system for either not treating, testing further (with either a rapid strep test or throat culture), or empirically treating with antibiotics.

Clinical question one

"Which physical examination findings alter the likelihood of a positive GAS culture in patients with a sore throat?"
A recent systematic review compiled data and calculated likelihood ratios (LR+ and LR−) for clinical findings and the chance of a positive GAS culture.[2] The following data is presented with respective 95% confidence intervals (CI): the most predictive elements included pharyngeal exudates [LR+ 2.1(1.4–3.1); LR− 0.90 (0.75–1.1)], tonsillar swelling/enlargement [LR+ 1.8 (1.5–2.3); LR− 0.63 (0.56–0.72)], tender anterior cervical nodes [LR+ (1.2–1.9); LR− 0.60 (0.49–0.71)], tonsillar exudates [LR+ 3.4 (1.8–6.0); LR- 0.72 (0.60–0.88)], no cough [LR+ (1.1–1.7); LR− (0.53–0.89)], and strep exposure within the previous two weeks [LR+ 1.9 (1.3–2.8); LR− 0.92 (0.86–0.99)]. Notably, no single clinical finding showed a good ability to discriminate through its presence or absence in GAS positive and negative patients with a sore throat.

Clinical question two

"What are the clinical prediction rules for GAS pharyngitis and how can they guide therapy for ED patients with a sore throat?"
The Centor criteria is a prediction rule based on selected signs and symptoms in patients with pharyngitis that can identify patients at low risk for GAS pharyngitis.[2] The Centor criteria include: (i) a history of fever; (ii) anterior cervical adenopathy; (iii) tonsillar exudates; and (iv) the absence of a cough. Using a positive culture for GAS as the gold standard, in the initial derivation study of the Centor criteria, probabilities assigned to each score included: a 56% probability of a positive culture in patients with four positive criteria, a 32% probability with three, a 15% probability with two, 6.5% with one, and 2.5% with no positive criteria.[3] The Centor criteria have since been validated in adult populations.

Given that the probability of a strep infection is higher in children because of the difference in the prevalence between adults and children, McIssac *et al.*

Table 22.1 The Centor strep score likelihood ratio (LR) and probability of infection from McIssac *et al.*[4]

Points	LR	Probability of infection
−1 or 0	0.05	1%
1	0.52	10%
2	0.95	17%
3	2.5	35%
4 or 5	4.9	51%

suggested a revision to the Centor criteria that would take age into account.[4] In the McIssac revision, if the patient was under five years old they would receive an additional point, whereas if they were over 45 years old they would have a point subtracted. Using the McIssac modification, the risk of streptococcal infection is listed in Table 22.1.

In each case, as we described in Chapter 2, a pre-test odds can be multiplied by the likelihood ratio, which in this instance would hence generate a post-test odds of GAS infection based on these criteria.

Comment

Specific signs and symptoms can increase or reduce the likelihood of patients with a sore throat having positive throat cultures for GAS. The Centor criteria with the McIssac modifications have been validated in both adults and children for use in predicting the probability of GAS pharyngitis. To determine the probability of GAS and the use of antibiotics, application of these criteria can be helpful in guiding testing and treatment decisions in the ED.

There is however, considerable controversy over how these rules should be applied in clinical practice and multiple management strategies have been suggested. Using two separate criteria as an example, the Infectious Disease Society of America (IDSA) and the American College of Physicians/American Society of Internal Medicine (ACP-ASIM) have proposed different management strategies for adults with pharyngitis (see Table 22.2).

The clinical balancing act centers on overtreatment (which may result in the inappropriate use of antibiotics for cases that are not a result of GAS) versus undertreatment (which may result in missed cases). It does make clinical sense given the higher prevalence of GAS pharyngitis in children to employ a liberal approach to testing, as per the IDSA guidelines in adults.

It should, however, be noted that the use of rapid strep tests is subject to spectrum bias, where there are different test sensitivities at different Centor scores (likelihoods of GAS pharyngitis).[6] According to this study, the Centor

Table 22.2 Adult pharyngitis guidelines for diagnostic testing and treatment with antibiotics (abx) based on the Centor score (adapted from Centor *et al.* 2007[5])

Centor score	Decision	IDSA	ACP-ASIM
0	Test	No	No
	Treat	No	No
1	Test	No	No
	Treat	No	No
2	Test	Rapid Strep	Rapid Strep
	Treat	Abx if rapid Strep+	Abx if rapid Strep+
3	Test	Rapid Strep	No test/rapid Strep
	Treat	Abx if rapid Strep+	Empirical abx/abx if Strep+
4	Test	Rapid Strep	No test
	Treat	Abx if rapid Strep+	Empirical abx

ACP-ASIM, American College of Physicians/American Society of Internal Medicine; IDSA, Infectious Disease Society of America.

score corresponded to the following rapid strep test sensitivities: Centor 0 or 1 = 61%; Centor 2 = 76%; Centor 3 = 90%; and Centor 4 = 97%. Given that rapid strep testing is not 100% sensitive, the recommendation of the American Academy of Pediatrics (AAP) is to culture all negative rapid strep tests. Given the number of negative tests, a recent guideline recommended by the AAP and the IDSA organizations was that EDs should consider validating locally that rapid strep tests are as sensitive as throat cultures.

References

1. Del Mar, C.B., Glasziou, P.P. and Spinks, A.B. (2003) Antibiotics for sore throat (Cochrane methodology review). In: *The Cochrane Library* **4**. John Wiley & Sons Ltd., Chicester, UK.

2. Ebell, M.H., Smith, M.A., Barry, H.C., *et al.* (2000) The rational clinical examination: does this patient have strep throat? *Journal of the American Medical Association* **284**: 2912–2918.

3. Centor, R., Witherspoon, J., Dalton, H., Brody, C. and Link, K. (1981) The diagnosis of strep throat in adults in the emergency room. *Medical Decision Making* **1**(3): 239–246.

4. McIsaac, W.J., Goel, V., To, T., *et al.* (2000) The validity of a sore throat score in family practice. *Canadian Medical Association Journal* **168**: 811–815.

5. Centor, R., Allison, J.J. and Cohen, S.J. (2007) Pharyngitis Management: Defining the Controvery. *Journal of General Internal Medical* **22**: 127–130.

6. DiMatteo, L.A., Lowenstein, S.R., Brimhall, B., *et al.* (2001) The relationship between the clinical features of pharyngitis and the sensitivity of a rapid antigen test: evidence of spectrum bias. *Annals of Emergency Medicine* **38**: 648–652.

Chapter 23 **Infective Endocarditis**

Highlights

- Infective endocarditis is a challenging diagnosis in the emergency department (ED).
- The major Duke criteria rely heavily on blood culture and echocardiography results.
- The minor Duke criteria provide risk factors that emergency physicians can use to stratify the risk of endocarditis.
- Transesophageal echocardiography is currently the superior method of evaluation for endocarditis because it is more sensitive in both native and prosthetic heart valves.

Background

Infective endocarditis is a microbial infection of the endocardial surface of the heart that has an incidence of between 1.8 and 7.0 per 100 000 people per year. Endocarditis is challenging to diagnose, primarily because of the presence of nonspecific clinical features at ED presentation. Because a missed diagnosis of endocarditis can lead to poor outcomes, emergency physicians must have a low threshold for the consideration of this potentially lethal disease. Fever is the most common symptom of endocarditis and some sources report that relapsing fevers lasting for a week or more should prompt consideration of this diagnosis. The second most common clinical feature is the presence of a murmur or evidence of valvular heart disease. Other common signs include splenomegaly, microscopic hematuria, anemia, and leukocytosis.

Over the past 30 years, there has been a shift in the epidemiology of endocarditis that has altered the prevalence of common classic cutaneous and

---

Evidence-Based Emergency Care: Diagnostic Testing and Clinical Decision Rules. By J.M. Pines and W.W. Everett. Published 2008 by Blackwell Publishing, ISBN: 978-14051-5400-0.

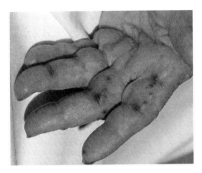

Figure 23.1 Janeway lesions from bacterial endocarditis. (Source: Wolff *et al. Fitzpatrick's Color Atlas and Synopsis of Clinical Dermatology* 4th Edition © 2001. Reproduced with permission of The McGraw-Hill Companies.)

ophthomologic manifestations such as Oslers nodes, Roth spots, Janeway lesions (Fig. 23.1), splinter hemorrhages, or oral petichiae.[1] These changes are primarily attributable to the increase in incidence of endocarditis in prosthetic valve recipients, intravenous drug abusers (IVDA), and geriatric patients.[2] There has also been a shift in the microbiology of endocarditis from primarily streptococci species to coagulase-positive and coagulase-negative staphylococci. This has led to a change in the classic presentation of infective endocarditis, where most commonly a patient with IVDA may present more acutely with right-sided valvular infections caused by *Staphalococcus aureus* without the classic peripheral stigmata of endocarditis.

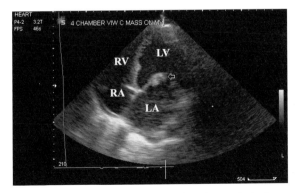

Figure 23.2 Apical four-chamber view demonstrating a large mitral valve vegetation (*arrow*). RA, right atrium; LA, left atrium; LV, left ventricle; RV, right ventricle. (Courtesy of Anthony Dean, MD.)

Clinical question

"What is the most accurate method of diagnosing suspected infective endocarditis in the ED?"

The best criteria for the diagnosis of endocarditis are the Duke criteria, which were initially suggested in 1994 by Dureck *et al.*[3] The Duke criteria were derived using 405 consecutive cases of suspected infective endocarditis in 353 patients between 1985 and 1992. The authors defined two 'major criteria' (positive blood culture and positive echocardiogram (Fig. 23.2)) and six 'minor criteria' (predisposition, fever, vascular phenomena, immunologic phenomena, suggestive echocardiogram, and suggestive microbiologic findings). They also defined three distinct diagnostic categories: 'definite' by pathologic or clinical criteria, 'possible,' and 'rejected.' A definite case was stated to be when there was direct evidence of infectious endocarditis based on histology or bacteriology of a vegetation or peripheral embolus. There were a total of 69 pathologically confirmed cases of definite endocarditis, and 55 (80%) of these were classified clinically as definite endocarditis. Table 23.1 provides a list of the Duke criteria.

Other studies have investigated how well the Duke criteria work in excluding a diagnosis of infective endocarditis. Dodd *et al.* investigated the long-term follow-up study of 49 episodes where there was suspected endocarditis but the diagnosis of endocarditis was rejected by the Duke criteria.[4] Of these, 63% had a firm alternative diagnosis established at the time of initial

Table 23.1 The Duke criteria for infective endocarditis (IE)

Criteria type	Diagnostic category	Criteria definitions
Pathologic	Definite IE	**Microorganisms**: demonstrated by culture or histology in a vegetation, in a vegetation that has embolized or in an intracardiac abscess or **Pathologic lesions**: vegetation or intracardiac abscess present, confirmed by histology showing active endocarditis
Clinical	Possible IE	Findings of endocarditis that fall short of definite, but not rejected
	Rejected (i.e. not IE)	Firm alternate diagnosis explaining evidence of IE or Resolution of endocarditis syndrome, with antibiotic therapy for ≤4 days or No pathologic evidence of IE at surgery or autopsy, after antibiotic therapy for ≤4 days

Table 23.1 (cont'd)

Criteria type	Diagnostic category	Criteria definitions
Major	Positive blood culture for IE	Typical microorganism for IE from 2 separate blood cultures: • viridans streptococci, *S. bovis*, or HACEK group or, • community-acquired *S. aureus* or enterococci, in the absence of a primary focus or Microorganism consistent with IE from persistently positive blood cultures. Either: • 2 positive cultures drawn >12 h apart, or • all or 3, or majority of 4 or more separate blood cultures, with first and last drawn at least 1 h apart
	Evidence of endocardial involvement	Positive echocardiogram for IE defined as: • oscillating intracardiac mass on valve or supporting structures, in the path of regurgitant jets, or on implanted material, in the absence of an alternative anatomic explanation, or • abscess, or • new partial dehiscence of a prosthetic valve or New valvular regurgitation (increase or change in pre-existing murmur not sufficient)
Minor	None	**Predisposition**: predisposing heart condition or intravenous drug use **Fever**: ≥38.0 C (100.4 F) **Vascular phenomena**: major arterial emboli, septic pulmonary infarcts, mycotic aneurysm, intracranial hemorrhage, conjunctival hemorrhages, and Janeway lesions **Immunologic phenomena**: glomerlonephritis, Osler's nodes, Roth spots, and rheumatoid factor **Echocardiographic findings**: consistent with IE but not meeting major criteria above **Microbiological evidence**: positive blood culture but not meeting major criteria

HACEK refers to a grouping of gram-negative bacilli: *Haemophilus* species (*H. parainfluenzae, H. aphrophilus,* and *H. paraphrophilus*), *Actinobacillus actinomycetemcomitans, Cardiobacterium hominis, Eikenella corrodens,* and *Kingella* species.

evaluation, 35% had syndromes that resolved spontaneously following four or fewer days of antibiotic treatment, and one patient had endocarditis ruled out at the time of heart surgery. Follow-up information was obtained for all patients at three months post-hospitalization. There was one patient who had a diagnosis of prosthetic-valve endocarditis and one patient who died, with a diagnosis of possible endocarditis on autopsy.

The Duke criteria have also been applied to a group of 100 patients with fever of unknown origin who had multiple blood cultures and who underwent echocardiography, in order to calculate the specificity of the criteria.[5] Similar to the study by Dodd *et al.*, 65% had an alternative diagnosis and 35% had a clinical syndrome that resolved after either short-term or no antibiotic therapy. There was only one patient who was misclassified as negative by the Duke criteria, making the criteria 99% specific.

Recently it has been proposed that the Duke criteria should be revised and the minor criteria, 'echocardiogram consistent with infective endocarditis,' eliminated as a result of the use of transesophageal echocardiography. There have been other recent suggestions for modifications, including adding further minor criteria, such as splenomegaly and a C-reactive protein (CRP) of 100 mg/L or above. In addition, other adjunctive testing, such as for procalcitonin levels, have been suggested to aid in the diagnosis of infective endocarditis. Mueller *et al.* performed a prospective cohort study in 67 patients admitted with the suspicion of infective endocarditis and inpatients with suspected endocarditis.[6] Infective endocarditis was diagnosed by the Duke criteria and confirmed in 21 patients. Procalcitonin levels were found to be higher in patients with endocarditis (median 6.56 ng/mL) than in those without (median 0.44 ng/mL, $P<0.001$). The optimal concentration of procalcitonin for calculating positive and negative predictive values was 2.3 ng/mL. With this cutoff, the test characteristics for procalcitonin were: sensitivity 81%, specificity 85%, negative predictive value 92%, and positive predictive value 72%.

The choice of echocardiograhic imaging technique has been the subject of controversy when comparing transthoracic echocardiography (TTE) to transesophageal echocardiography (TEE). Because in TEE the transducer is in much closer proximity to the heart, there is an improved ability to visualize smaller structures including small vegetations, leaflet perforations, and small (<5 mm) abscesses. TEE is currently the superior method of evaluation for endocarditis as it is more sensitive in both native and prosthetic heart valves.

Comment

In the context of the diagnosis of endocarditis in the ED, the major microbiological Duke criteria cannot be met on initial evaluation unless blood cultures are drawn in advance. Patients may be evaluated for endocarditis by the use of a TTE or a TEE. A TEE in the ED is technically more challenging because it requires sedation. Echocardiograms are also not a commonly ordered ED test unless the patient is unstable or an emergent echocardiogram is guiding ED management. Even in emergency cases, some hospital EDs may have limited access to echocardiography.

However, emergency echocardiograms can change the management of a patient within the ED, particularly in the presence of an intracardiac abscess. The most common life-threatening complication of infective endocarditis is congestive heart failure, with the most common cause being infection-induced valvular damage. Because heart failure is a common ED presentation, infective endocarditis should be considered in patients with new murmurs and acute congestive heart failure in an appropriate clinical setting (i.e. where other risk factors such as IVDA are present).

While TEE is the current recommended test for ruling out endocarditis, particularly for patients with suspected, complicated infective endocarditis and for patients with suspected prosthetic valve endocarditis, this may be even more difficult to order in the ED than a traditional TTE.[7] Procalcitonin levels may be helpful in diagnosing endocarditis in the ED; however, procalcitonin levels may also be difficult to order on an emergency basis, depending upon the laboratory. C-reactive protein levels may be easier to order on an emergency basis, but these are relatively nonspecific. Because blood cultures are the most important laboratory diagnostic test in suspected endocarditis and can provide antibiotic suspectibility results that can guide long-term treatment, the current recommendation is to draw three sets of blood cultures.

The Duke minor criteria provide factors by which an emergency physician may stratify risk of endocarditis. The presence of a predisposing heart condition such as rheumatic heart disease, valvular heart disease or other abnormalities, or IVDA should raise suspicion for endocarditis in the context of a fever or other symptoms of infection. Other risk factors include indwelling catheters and patients on long-term hemodialysis; other considerations in the evaluation of infective endocarditis include the presence of a previously undocumented heart murmur. Vascular phenomenon and immunologic phenomenon should be evaluated on physical examination in these patients as these are minor criteria. However, given the change in the microbiology and epidemiology of endocarditis over the past 30 years, these types of lesions are less frequently seen. Some thought should also be given to including the presence of leukocytosis, microscopic hematuria, and anemia in the evaluation of suspected endocarditis, as these are commonly ordered tests and may be present in endocarditis.

References

1. Bayer, A.S. (1996) Diagnosis and management of infectious endocarditis. *Cardiology Clinical* **14**(3): 345–351.
2. Bayer, A.S. (1993) Infectious endocarditis: state of the art. *Clinical Infectious Diseases* **17**: 313–322.
3. Dureck, D.T., Lukes, A.S. and Bright, D.K. and the Duke Endocarditis Service. (1994) New criteria for diagnosis of infective endocarditis: utilization of specific echocardiographic findings. *American Journal of Medicine* **96**(3): 200–209.
4. Dodds, G.A. III, Sexton, D.J., Durack, D.T., *et al.* and the Duke Endocarditis Service. (1996) Negative predictive value of the Duke criteria for infective endocarditis. *American Journal of Cardiology* **77**: 403–407.
5. Hoen, B., Beguinot, I., Maignan, M., *et al.* (1996) The Duke criteria for the diagnosis of infective endocarditis are specific: An analysis of 100 patients with acute fever or fever of unknown origin. *Clinical Infectious Diseases* **23**(2): 298–302.
6. Mueller, C., Huber, P., Laifer, G., *et al.* (2004) Procalcitonin and the early diagnosis of endocarditis. *Circulation* **109**: 1707–1710.
7. Horstkotte, D., Follath, F., Gutschik, E., *et al.* (2004) Guidelines on prevention, diagnosis and treatment of infective endocarditis – executive summary. *European Heart Journal* **25**: 267–276.

Chapter 24 **Urinary Tract Infection**

Highlights

- Urinary tract infections (UTIs) commonly affect young women and older men with disorders of the prostate.
- Urine culture is the gold standard for UTIs and results are not available at the time of emergency department (ED) care.
- Urine dipsticks are not highly sensitive indicators of positive urine cultures; however, information from the urine dipstick can be used in conjunction with clinical pre-test probability.
- Because UTI symptoms and dipstick testing are not highly sensitive and specific, patients should receive a full examination (including pelvic examinations), especially if vaginal symptoms are present.

Background

Urinary tract infections (UTI) are common complaints in emergency medicine practice. Young women account for most of the seven million UTIs per year. UTIs are relatively uncommon in young men and tend to affect older men and be associated with disorders of the prostate. The most common way to diagnose UTIs in the ED is via either a urine dipstick test, which measures urinary leukocytes, nitrite, blood, protein, and pH, or laboratory urinalysis.

The diagnosis of UTI can be difficult in the ED because of the often inconsistent relationship between the clinical symptoms, bacteriuria and pyuria. In addition, because the gold standard test (urine culture) cannot be completed in the ED because it can take 2–3 days to grow, emergency physicians must diagnose and treat UTIs without gold standard testing. There are problems

Evidence-Based Emergency Care: Diagnostic Testing and Clinical Decision Rules. By J.M. Pines and W.W. Everett. Published 2008 by Blackwell Publishing, ISBN: 978-14051-5400-0.

with both overtreatment and misdiagnosis of UTIs in EDs and ambulatory settings given the common complaints and multiple alternative etiologies (i.e. vaginal or cervical infections).

Clinical question one

"What is the sensitivity and specificity of urine dipstick and urinalysis for diagnosing urinary tract infections in the ED?"

There are many studies that have directly addressed this question. We describe two relevant studies in this chapter. Semeniuk and Church evaluated the use of leukocyte esterase and nitrite as screening tests for the detection of bacteriuria in women with suspected uncomplicated urinary tract infections in a non-ED setting.[1] Subsequently, Lammers *et al.* published a study investigating the test characteristics of urine dipstick and urinalysis in ED and intermediate care patients.[2]

The paper by Semeniuk and Church reported data on 479 women and sought to determine the sensitivity and specificity as well as the predictive values for urinalysis, as compared with differing quantitative cutoffs, for defining a positive urine culture [i.e. 10^3–10^5 colony-forming units (CFU)/mL]. The highest sensitivities for urinalysis were demonstrated with the presence of both nitrite and leukocyte esterase (84%), and with leukocyte esterase alone (84%), at a cutoff of 10^5 CFU/mL. Interestingly, the presence of leukocyte esterase alone had a very low positive predictive value (PPV) at all CFU cutoffs (3–19%), while the PPVs of nitrite and leukocyte esterase together or nitrite alone were higher (84% and 75%, respectively), using a cutoff of 10^5 CFU/mL. The negative predictive values (NPVs) were all very high for the absence of any leukocyte esterase or nitrite, with values ranging from 97–99%. This study concluded that women with urinary tract symptoms can have low levels of bactiuria (less than 10^5 CFU/mL), and that this may represent urethral colonization. They also highlighted the fact that 19% of positive cultures with significant bacteriuria (>10^5 CFU/mL) would have been missed if a urine culture had not been ordered.

Lammers *et al.* carried out a prospective, observational study investigating the test characteristics of both urine dipstick and urinalysis using multiple test cutoff points in females with symptoms of a UTI (dysuira, urgency, or urinary frequency on history, or suprapubic or costovertebral angle tenderness on examination) who were seen in the ED and an intermediate care center. They excluded patients who had taken antibiotics within the previous 72 h, or who had indwelling Foley cathethers, symptomatic vaginal discharge, diabetes, or human immunodeficiency virus (HIV). A positive urine culture in this study was treated as the gold standard; this was defined as having more than 10^5 CFU/mL of one or two uropathogenic bacteria at 48 h after collection. In 349 patients, a little less than half had positive cultures. Urine dipstick results were defined as positive when either nitrite or leukocyte esterase were positive, or when blood was more than trace; the overtreatment rate was 47% (defined as 1–PPV) and the undertreatment rate was 13%. By defining a positive urinalysis as having more than three white blood cells per high power field, or when red blood cells were in excess of five per high power field, the overtreatment rate was 44% and the undertreatment rate was 11%. The authors concluded that similar overtreatment and undertreatment rates were identified for various test cutoff points for urine dipstick tests and urinalysis.

Clinical question two

"How does the addition of clinical symptoms augment the predictive value for urine dipsticks?"

One study originating from the UK directly addressed this question.[3] Little and colleagues sought to estimate dipstick and clinical predictors of UTI in a primary care setting. They studied 429 women with symptoms of UTI and used a low cutoff (10^3 CFU/mL) as the gold standard. They found that nitrite, leukocyte esterase and blood (trace or greater) independently predicted the presence of UTIs with respective odds ratios of 6.36, 4.52, and 2.23. A dipstick-only decision rule, which included having either nitrite or leukocyte esterase and blood, was 77% sensitive and 70% specific, with a PPV of 81% and an NPV of 65%. If all three were negative, the NPV was 73%. A clinical decision rule was derived based on having two of the following symptoms: urine cloudiness, an offensive smell, and dysuria and/or noctiuria of moderate severity, with sensitivity 65%, specificity 69%, PPV 77%, and NPV 54%. NPV was 71% if there were no clinical features and PPV was 84% if three or more symptoms were present. Interestingly, the performance of the clinical prediction rule was not improved by adding together both the dipstick and clinical results. The authors were also concerned that their data differed considerably with regard to NPVs for leukocyte esterease, nitrite, and blood, with reported NPVs in the range 50–70% compared to values approaching 90–100% in other studies.

Comment

This chapter highlights the continued difficulty in identifying ED patients with UTIs without gold standard testing information available at the point of care (i.e. urine culture). In the context of clinical ED practice, this short review identifies a number of conclusions and observations from the literature for the care of females with suspected UTIs. First, the performances of urinary dipstick tests and urinalysis were similar in the paper by Lammers *et al.* and were shown to be not highly sensitive. While one paper should not necessarily change practice, this indicates that a point of care urine dipstick may be a reasonable diagnostic endpoint in a classic presentation of UTI (i.e. high pre-test probability). Also, the absence of leukocyte esterase, nitrite, and blood does not fully exclude UTI. Clinical judgment and patient resources should be balanced when deciding to treat patients with negative tests and classic symptoms. One caveat to consider when reviewing these studies is that the authors described the use of dipsticks in what were effectively ideal clinical settings where patients with vaginal complaints were excluded. In ED practice a full evaluation, including a pelvic examination, should be performed on women with any vaginal symptoms, even in the absence of a positive dipstick test.

References

1. Semeniuk, H. and Church, D. (1999) Evaluation of the leukocyte esterase and nitrite urine dipstick screening tests for detection of bactiuria in women with suspected uncomplicated urinary tract infections. *Journal of Clinical Microbiology* **37**: 3051–3052.
2. Lammers, R.L., Gibson, S., Kovacs, D., *et al.* (2001) Comparison of test characteristics of urine dipstick and urinalysis at various test cutoff points. *Annals of Emergency Medicine* **38**: 505–512.
3. Little, P., Turner, S., Rumsby, K., *et al.* (2006) Developing clinical rules to predict urinary tract infections in primary care settings: sensitivity and specificity of near patient tests (dipsticks) and clinical scores. *British Journal of General Practice* **56**(529): 606–612.

Chapter 25 **Sinusitis**

Highlights

- The vast majority of patients with symptoms of sinus congestion in the emergency department (ED) will have viral infections.
- The gold standard for the diagnosis of bacterial sinusitis is sinus puncture, which is not practical in the ED.
- Sinus imaging has been used as a gold standard in some studies, but sinus imaging is not currently recommended in the ED unless invasive disease is suspected.
- Certain clinical symptoms and signs are suggestive of acute bacterial sinusitis including a 'double sickening', length of symptoms >10 days, unilateral facial pain, mucopurulent nasal discharge, unilateral maxillary tenderness, and maxillary toothache.
- A Task Force on Rhinosinusitis has stratified the diagnosis of acute bacterial sinusitis on the basis of at least two major factors (facial pain/pressure, facial congestion/fullness, nasal obstruction, nasal purulence or discolored postnasal discharge, hyposmia or anosmia, or fever), or one major and two minor factors (headache, halitosis, fatigue, dental pain, cough, ear pain, pressure, fullness, or fever). The validity of this recommendation has not been tested.

Background

The complaint of sinus congestion is very common in emergency care. The majority of patients with such complaints have viral infections while a small subset will have acute bacterial sinusitis, requiring treatment with antibiotics. Acute bacterial sinusitis is typically preceded by a viral upper respiratory tract

Evidence-Based Emergency Care: Diagnostic Testing and Clinical Decision Rules. By J.M. Pines and W.W. Everett. Published 2008 by Blackwell Publishing, ISBN: 978-14051-5400-0.

infection, and less commonly by allergic rhinitis. Approximately 0.5–2% of cases of acute viral upper respiratory tract infections will be complicated by acute bacterial sinusitis in adults, while in children the proportion is considerably higher at 6–13%. Therefore, differentiating patients who present with symptoms of sinus inflammation caused by viral or allergic causes compared with bacterial causes is a clinical challenge for emergency and primary care physicians. The gold standard diagnosis for acute bacterial sinusitis is sinus puncture and culture, both of which are impractical in the ED setting. Sinus imaging has been used in some studies as a gold standard. However, imaging is not 100% accurate; in many cases sinus imaging can be positive and the sinusitis can still be of viral etiology. Currently sinus imaging is not recommended for patients unless more invasive disease (i.e. orbital) is suspected.

Clinical question

"Which clinical features are associated with acute bacterial sinusitis in ambulatory ED patients?"

Given the absence of a sensitive ED-based test for sinusitis, the diagnosis of acute bacterial sinusitis and the decision to treat with antibiotics is often made on clinical grounds based on the history and physical examination. A strong factor in distinguishing patients with acute bacterial sinusitis is the duration of symptoms. One trial studied the natural course of rhinosinusitis and found that 60% of patients who reported symptoms persisting for at least 10 days had a positive bacterial culture from a sinus aspirate. On that basis, consensus groups have recommended different time intervals for making a diagnosis of acute bacterial sinusitis and for subsequent antibiotic therapy. Some groups recommend seven days of symptoms as an appropriate time to use antibiotics, others have recommended that antibiotics should be withheld for up to ten days in children. This recommendation was based on a study of 2013 children, which found that of those screened at 10 days with Waters view radiography, 92% had a confirmed radiographic diagnosis of sinusitis.[1] Other recommendations include only treating if there is a worsening of the patient's clinical status after five to six days, regardless of the overall duration of the illness.

Studies of the signs and symptoms of sinusitis are limited by the choice of a gold standard. There are no studies to date that have used the gold standard of growth of 10^5 CFU/mL or greater from a sinus aspirate. Those reported have varied considerably in their use of a gold standard, from purulent sinus aspirates to sinus radiography. One early study (from 1988) evaluated 155 patients with acute sinusitis and found that unilateral purulent nasal discharge, unilateral facial pain, physical examination findings of purulent nasal discharge, and pus in the nasal cavity were the predominant symptoms to be highly associated with a positive radiography for sinusitis. They calculated a sensitivity of 81% and a specificity of 88% in patients with three or four of these signs or symptoms.[2]

Another study of 247 men with rhinorrhea, facial pain, or self-suspected sinusitis in the Veterans Health Administration system in the US used plain radiography as the gold standard and found five independent predictors of sinusitis: (i) maxillary toothache [odds ratio (OR): 2.9]; (ii) lack of transillumination (OR: 2.7); (iii) poor response to nasal decongestants or antihistamines (OR: 2.4); (iv) report of colored nasal discharge (OR: 2.2); and (v) purulent mucus on physical examination (OR: 2.9).[3]

Another paper used computed tomography (CT) findings as the gold standard and studied 201 patients with clinically diagnosed acute sinusitis.[4] More than half met the CT criteria for acute bacterial sinusitis (i.e. an air-fluid level or total opacification of any sinus) (Fig. 25.1). Four signs or symptoms were independently (and significantly) associated with a CT diagnosis of bacterial sinusitis: (i) purulent nose secretion; (ii) purulent rhinorrhea; (iii) 'double sickening' (defined as the presence of two phases of illness history); and (iv) an erythrocyte sedimentation rate of greater than 10 mm/h. The presence of three or more of these yielded a sensitivity of 66% and a specificity of 81%. The authors felt that 'double sickening,' which had an

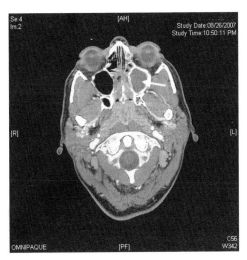

Figure 25.1 Head computed tomography showing sinusitis with left maxillary occlusion (arrow).

OR of 2.8, was particularly relevant given the association with the natural history of a viral upper respiratory infection followed by a secondary bacterial infection. This study also found that 82% of patients with CT-confirmed sinusitis had symptoms for 10 or more days, while 74% without CT findings had symptoms of less than seven days duration.

A more recent study used three separate gold standards in 174 adult patients with suspected sinusitis: CT, sinus aspiration, and culture.[5] Of the 70% with abnormal CT findings, only half met the diagnostic criteria for acute bacterial sinusitis (i.e. the presence of a purulent or mucopurulent sinus aspirate). Signs and symptoms associated with a positive culture included unilateral facial pain (OR: 1.9), maxillary toothache (OR: 1.9), unilateral maxillary tenderness (OR: 2.5), and mucopurulent nasal discharge (OR: 1.6).

Taken together these results suggest that acute bacterial sinusitis may be characterized by the clinical signs and symptoms of: (i) unilateral facial pain; (ii) mucopurulent nasal discharge; (iii) unilateral maxillary tenderness; and (iv) maxillary toothache. No single clinical finding is sensitive and specific enough to diagnose acute bacterial sinusitis. The Task Force on Rhinosinusitis of the American Academy of Otolaryngology-Head and Neck Surgery has provided guidance by stratifying specific diagnostic factors into major and minor categories.[6] They have stratified the diagnosis of acute bacterial sinusitis on the basis of at least two major factors (facial pain/pressure, facial congestion/fullness, nasal obstruction, nasal purulence or discolored postnasal discharge, hyposmia or anosmia, or fever), or one major and two minor factors (headache, halitosis, fatigue, dental pain, cough, ear pain, pressure, fullness, or fever). The validity of this classification system is based not on culture results of sinus aspirates but on sinus imaging, which is not a validated gold standard.

Comment

The diagnosis of acute bacterial sinusitis in the ED setting is a challenge due to the absence of an empirically validated decision rule to identify which patients to treat. Clinical signs and symptoms, duration of illness, and patient resources must be considered in determining which patients should be treated. Guidelines regarding the treatment of acute bacterial sinusitis are primarily based on the literature discussed in this chapter and on expert consensus. However, in comparison to the primary care setting, as ED physicians we frequently will not see the patients in follow-up, so a plan for close follow-up may not be feasible in all of our patients. One potential management strategy may be to write a prescription for patients with clinical signs and symptoms suspicious for sinusitis with explicit recommendations to fill the prescription if symptoms do not remit for seven days. However, using this strategy in clinical ED practice has not been validated empirically.

References

1. Ueda, D. and Yoto, Y. (1996) The ten-day mark as a practical diagnostic approach for acute paranasal sinusitis in children. *Pediatric Infectious Disease Journal* **15**: 576–579.
2. Berg, O. and Carenfelt, C. (1988) Analysis of symptoms and clinical signs in the maxillary sinus empyema. *Acta Oto-laryngologica* **105**: 343–349.
3. Williams, J.W., Jr, Simel, D.L., Roberts, L., *et al.* (1992) Clinical evaluation for sinusitis: making the diagnosis by history and physical examination. *Annals of Internal Medicine* **117**: 705–710.
4. Lindbaek, M., Hjortdahl, P. and Johnsen, U.L. (1996) Use of symptoms, signs, and blood tests to diagnose acute sinus infections in primary care: comparison with computed tomography. *Family Medicine* **28**: 183–188.
5. Hansen, J.G., Schmidt, H., Rosborg, J., *et al.* (1995) Predicting acute maxillary sinusitis in a general practice population. *British Medical Journal* **311**: 233–236.
6. Brooks, I., Gooch, W.M., III, Jenkins, S.G., *et al.* (2000) Medical management of acute bacterial sinusitis: recommendations of a clinical advisory committee on pediatric and adult sinusitis. *Annals of Otology, Rhinology and Laryngology* **182**(Suppl): 2–20.

Chapter 26 **Pneumonia**

Highlights

- The Pneumonia Severity Index (PSI) accurately discriminates patients at low risk for 30-day mortality.
- The CURB-65 rule accurately stratifies patients at high risk for 30-day mortality.
- A combination of these risk stratification tools and clinical judgment can be used when making disposition decisions for emergency department (ED) patients with pneumonia.

One of the challenges when evaluating patients in the ED with community-acquired pneumonia (CAP) (Fig. 26.1) is the assessment of illness severity, which in this disease will often guide decisions about admission, further diagnostic testing, and the choice of antibiotics. Several scoring systems have been developed to aid in ED decision making regarding patients with CAP.

Probably the most widely used scoring system is the PSI, which was developed by Fine *et al.*[1] Tables 26.1 and 26.2 detail the elements of the PSI and demonstrate that the PSI is associated with risk of death at 30 days. The primary purpose of the PSI was to identify patients who were at low risk for mortality and could be managed on an outpatient basis (i.e. at home). The authors have suggested that groups I, II, and III have mortality rates that are sufficiently low, and that these groups could therefore be treated as outpatients.

The CURB-65 score was developed by the British Thoracic Society. The purpose of CURB-65 is to identify patients that are at high risk of mortality from pneumonia. The following list includes the elements of the CURB-65 scoring system; each element is assigned one point when positive:

Evidence-Based Emergency Care: Diagnostic Testing and Clinical Decision Rules. By J.M. Pines and W.W. Everett. Published 2008 by Blackwell Publishing, ISBN: 978-14051-5400-0.

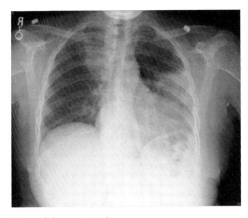

Figure 26.1 Left lower lobe pneumonia.

Table 26.1 The Pneumonia Severity Index from Fine *et al.*[1]

Characteristic	Points assigned
Demographic factor:	
Men	Age (years)
Women	Age (years) –10
Nursing-home resident	+10
Co-existing illnesses:	
Neoplastic disease	+30
Liver disease	+20
Congestive heart failure	+10
Cerebrovascular disease	+10
Renal disease	+10
Physical examination findings:	
Altered mental status	+20
Respiratory rate 30 breaths/min	+20
Systolic blood pressure <90 mmHg	+20
Temperature <35°C (95°F) or 40°C (104°F)	+15
Pulse 125 bpm	+10
Laboratory and radiographic findings (if study performed):	
Arterial blood pH <7.35	+30
Blood urea nitrogen level 30 mg/dL	+20
Sodium level <130 mmol/L	+20
Glucose level 250 mg/dL	+10
Hematocrit <30%	+10
Partial pressure of arterial 02 <60 mm Hg or 02 Sat <90%	+10
Pleural effusion	+10

Table 26.2 The Pneumonia Severity Index: classification according to points score from Fine et al.[1]

Class	Points	Mortality
I	<51	0.1%
II	51–70	0.6%
III	71–90	0.9%
IV	91–130	9.5%
V	>130	26.7%

- confusion;
- elevated blood urea nitrogen (BUN; >7 mmol/L);
- respiratory rate ($\geq$30/min);
- blood pressure (systolic <90 mmHg or diastolic $\leq$60 mmHg); and
- age $\geq$65 years.

Mortalities for the six-point scores found in an international derivation and validation study were 0.7% for score 0, 3.2% for score 1, 3% for score 2, 17% for score 3, 41.5% for score 4, and 57% for score 5.

The authors of the CURB-65 criteria have suggested that patients who score 0 or 1 are at low risk for mortality and can be managed as outpatients, those who have a score of 2 have an intermediate risk, and those with scores greater than 2 have severe CAP and are at high risk and hence should be managed in an intensive care unit.

Clinical question one

"Which severity adjustment tool provides the best discriminatory power in predicting survival in patients with pneumonia?"

A recent study compared the PSI to CURB-65 in 3181 ED patients.[2] Both the PSI and CURB-65 were good predictors of 30-day mortality and were also good at identifying patients at low risk of mortality. However, the PSI appeared to be better at identifying patients with a lower risk of mortality. Using the PSI, 68% were identified as low risk (class I–III) with a mortality rate of 1.4%, while CURB-65 identified 61% as low risk (score 0 or 1) with a mortality rate of 1.7%. In more severe CAP (score $\geq$2) CURB-65 seemed to be of greater use because each score (2–5) was associated with a progressive increase in mortality, while the PSI only discriminated between high-risk and low-risk groups.

Another study used the PSI and CURB-65 in a large group of both inpatients and outpatients with CAP in Spain.[3] The authors found that both CURB-65 and CRB-65 (a simpler version that excludes the BUN measurement) accurately predicted 30-day mortality rate, mechanical ventilation, and to some degree, hospitalization. CURB-65 also correlated with time to clinical stability and was predictive of a longer duration of intravenous antibiotics. The PSI also predicted mortality well in this study.

Clinical question two

"Can procalcitonin be used to predict survival in pneumonia and a bacterial etiology of infection?"
One study followed 185 patients who had procalcitonin levels measured within 24 h of admission for CAP.[4] The authors found that procalcitonin levels correlated with the PSI score and also predicted complications including the development of empyema, the need for mechanical ventilation, septic shock, and mortality. An interesting finding of this study was that a low PSI score predicted a bacterial etiology for pneumonia. These findings did not apply to those with more severe CAP.

Comment

The two major scoring systems for severity of illness in CAP—PSI and CURB-65—have been widely studied. The PSI seems to be a more reliable way of identifying patients that have a low risk of mortality. However, there is a tendency for the PSI to underestimate the severity of illness in younger patients with comorbid illness because it places a heavy weight on age and comoribidities. CURB-65 seems to be somewhat better at identifying patients that are at a higher risk for mortality and discriminates better among the more severely ill patients. One problem with CURB-65 is that it does not account as well for comorbidities. It also may be difficult to use in older patients with other chronic conditions who are at high risk for mortality, even though they may have a lower CURB-65 score.

While both scoring systems seem to be good tools for predicting survival in CAP, neither is perfect for differentiating which patients can be safely admitted or discharged from the ED. Other factors including clinical and social variables, and having adequate access to follow-up health care visits must be factored into this decision.

A recent commentary has suggested that the PSI and CURB-65 be combined, and this report also recognized that each system has its own limitations.[5] The authors suggested that low-risk patients (PSI class I–III or CURB-65 score 0–1) could be managed at home if serious vital sign abnormalities and comorbidities were absent, as measured by both scoring systems, and if no other factors (such as social situation) necessitated hospital admission.

Finally, procalcitonin may be a promising tool for predicting survival in patients with CAP. In addition, it may be helpful in guiding decisions regarding the use of antibiotics in lower risk patients. However, before it is used in ED patients to guide antibiotic decisions, larger studies must be performed.

References

1. Fine, M.J., Auble, T.E., Yealy, D.M., et al. (1997) A prediction rule to identify low-risk patients with community-acquired pneumonia. *New England Journal of Medicine* **336**: 243–250.
2. Aujesky, D., Auble, T.E., Yealy, D.M. et al. (2005) Prospective comparison of three validated prediction rules for prognosis in community-acquired pneumonia. *American Journal of Medicine* **118**: 384–392.
3. Capelastegui, A., Espana, P.P., Quintana, J.M., et al. (2006) Validation of a predictive rule for the management of community-acquired pneumonia. *European Respiratory Journal* **27**: 151–157.
4. Masia, M., Gutierrez, F., Shum, C., et al. (2005) Usefulness of procalcitonin levels in community-acquired pneumonia according to the patients outcome research team pneumonia severity index. *Chest* **128**: 2223–2229.
5. Niederman, M.S., Feldman, C. and Richards, G.A. (2006) Combining information from prognostic scoring tools for CAP: an American view on how to get the best of all worlds. *European Respiratory Journal* **27**: 9–11.

Chapter 27 **Spontaneous Bacterial Peritonitis**

Highlights

- Diagnosing spontaneous bacterial peritonitis (SBP) requires a paracentesis to sample the peritoneal fluid.
- Missing the diagnosis of SBP carries a high risk of mortality.
- Formal analysis and culture of the peritoneal fluid should be routinely performed when SBP is suspected.
- Rapid colorimetric reagent strips commonly used in dipstick testing of urine are highly sensitive in confirming a diagnosis of SBP.

Background

Spontaneous bacterial peritonitis (SBP) is an infection of the usually sterile intra-abdominal cavity involving ascitic fluid. SBP occurs in patients with hepatic disease, most commonly cirrhosis. The prevalence in unselected hospitalized cirrhotic patients ranges from 10 to 30%. Mortality from SBP has improved with aggressive empiric antibiotic treatment but still remains high at around 30%. By definition, the source of the intra-abdominal infection is uncertain, making reliance on the history and physical examination important in order to consider the diagnosis. Ultimately though, sampling of the ascitic fluid via paracentesis is required (Fig. 27.1). The diagnosis of SBP requires a polymorphonuclear (PMN) cell count of above 250/mL in the ascitic fluid to start empiric antibiotic treatment; however, the diagnosis can also be made with cell counts below 250/mL if an organism is identified from cultures of the ascitic fluid. Despite efforts to identify both the organism and the source of the infection, cultures of ascitic fluid yield an organism in roughly 40–50% of cases. In addition, there is not always immediate access

Evidence-Based Emergency Care: Diagnostic Testing and Clinical Decision Rules. By J.M. Pines and W.W. Everett. Published 2008 by Blackwell Publishing, ISBN: 978-14051-5400-0.

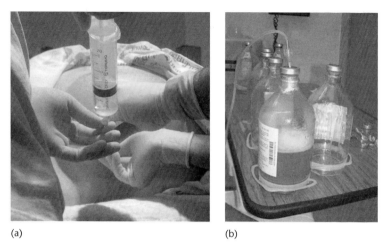

(a)   (b)

Figure 27.1 (a) Needle aspiration of ascites during a paracentesis. (b) When there is ample fluid, larger volumes of ascitic fluid can be removed.

to a good and reliable laboratory for testing, emergent cell counts can be delayed, and cultures can take days to grow. Therefore, alternative methods for the rapid diagnosis of SBP have been sought.

Clinical question

"Can rapid colorimetric reagent strips commonly used in urine dipstick testing be used with ascitic fluid to accurately diagnose SBP?"

Leukocyte esterase (LE) reacts with a chemical compound strip to produce a colorimetric change that is proportional to the concentration of the LE in the sample, and hence the number of PMNs present. This reaction has been used commonly in the assessment of urine, but the principle is the same for measuring LE levels in any bodily fluid. Urine strips are commonly found in emergency departments (EDs) and acute care settings and are easy to use. Several studies have examined the applicability of such 'urine dipsticks' to ascitic fluid for the rapid assessment of SBP.

At least three recent studies have examined the usefulness of rapid reagent strips for diagnosing SBP in patients with hepatic disease. The earliest of these was carried out by Spanish scientists who examined ascitic fluid in unselected cirrhotic patients admitted to a university-based hospital.[1] Following the paracentesis, ascitic fluid was tested using a commercially available urine reagent strip (Aution sticks®, A. Menarini Diagnostics, Firenze, Italy). The five-grade colorimetric scale is linearly correlated to the PMN counts (grades

Table 27.1 Test characteristics of a reagent strip (Aution stick®) for detecting spontaneous bacterial peritonitis (SBP) from Castellote *et al.*[1]

	SBP (+)	SBP (−)	Total
Reagent strip grade 3 or 4 (+)	51	1	52
Reagent strip grades 0, 1, or 2 (−)	6	170	176
Total	57	171	228
Sensitivity, % (95% CI)		89 (81–97)	
Specificity, % (95% CI)		99 (98–100)	
PPV, % (95% CI)		98 (94–100)	
NPV, % (95% CI)		97 (94–100)	
Diagnostic accuracy, % (95% CI)		97 (95–99)	

NPV, negative predictive value; PPV, positive predictive value.

0–4 are equivalent to a PMN count of 0, 25, 75, 250, and 500/mL, respectively). Two investigators, blinded to each other's results, rated the strip at 90 sec. The test was considered positive if the reagent strip was grade 3 or 4, corresponding to a PMN count of 250/mL or higher. The gold standard was a PMN count of 250/mL or above in the ascitic fluid, as determined by the hospital laboratory.

A total of 228 paracentesis in 128 patients were included. A diagnosis of SBP was made in 52 cases, with 23 (44%) of these yielding positive ascitic fluid cultures. Table 27.1 shows the performance characteristics of the reagent strip. The authors concluded that the rapid assessment of ascitic fluid using a colorimetric scale with a commonly available chemical reagent strip could be useful in the rapid diagnosis of SBP.

Korean researchers studied 53 consecutive cirrhotic patients hospitalized over a six month period in 2003 and 2004.[2] Using similar methods to those reported in the previous study, the ascitic fluid was tested using two kinds of urine strips (UriSCAN®, Young-Dong Corp., Seoul, Korea; Multistix10SG®, Bayer Corp., Bridgend, UK). The UriSCAN has a four-grade scale (0–3) corresponding to PMN counts of 0, 25, 75, and 500/mL, respectively. The Multistix10SG has a five-grade scale (0–4) corresponding to PMN counts of 0–4, 5–9, 10–29, 30–74, and 75–200/mL, respectively. The UriSCAN test was performed in all paracentesis cases (n = 75), while the Multistix10SG was available for only 62 of the 75 cases.

Overall there were 18 cases of SBP (incidence 24%). When the UriSCAN was considered positive with a grade of three or above, the sensitivity, specificity, positive predictive value (PPV), negative predictive value (NPV), and accuracy were 67%, 100%, 100%, 89%, and 91%, respectively. If the

UriSCAN was considered positive with a grade of two or above, then all performance parameters were 100%.

In comparison, if the Multistix10SG was considered positive with a grade of three or above, the test had a sensitivity, specificity, PPV, NPV, and accuracy 50%, 100%, 100%, 87%, and 89%, respectively. The authors concluded that although the sample size of the study was small and all patients were hospitalized, both reagent strips were highly accurate.

A French study examined 245 ascitic samples from 51 patients using two chemical reagent strips for quantifying LE (Nephur-Test®, Roche diagnostics, Meylan, France; and Multistix10SG®).[3] For this study, any colorimetric change on the reagent strip was considered a positive test. Inter-rater reliability was assessed between a study physician and a non-study nurse; these results were then compared to the gold standard of standard laboratory reported cell counts. There were 17 cases of SBP in this study, yielding a prevalence of 7%. The sensitivity, specificity, PPV, NPV, and accuracy of each test are shown in Table 27.2. There was 100% agreement in the reagent test strip readings obtained by the physician and the nurse.

The authors concluded that both reagent strips were sufficiently accurate to warrant consideration for clinical use in ambulatory settings where laboratory facilities may not be available. However, given the low occurrence of disease in this study, larger studies are needed in order to determine which strip is superior and whether the test performances are of a high enough standard to forgo formal laboratory analysis other than culture.

Comments

It is recommended that patients with ascites that is of recent onset or is resistant/refractory to medical therapy undergo an 'exploratory' paracentesis. Missing the diagnosis of SBP carries with it a high risk of mortality, which

Table 27.2 A comparison of the sensitivity of two separate reagent strips for detecting spontaneous bacterial peritonitis from Sapey et al.[3]

	Nephur-Test® (n = 245)	Multistix10SG® (n = 245)
Sensitivity, % (95% CI)	88 (62–98)	65 (39–85)
Specificity, % (95% CI)	100 (97–100)	100 (97–100)
PPV, % (95% CI)	94 (68–100)	92 (60–100)
NPV, % (95% CI)	99 (96–100)	97 (94–99)
Diagnostic accuracy, % (95% CI)	99 (96–100)	97 (94–99)

NPV, negative predictive value; PPV, positive predictive value.

remains as high as 20–30% even when appropriate antibiotic treatment is administered. Once considered, the diagnosis of SBP requires a paracentesis along with a formal laboratory analysis and culture of the ascitic fluid.

The three studies described above have examined different colorimetric chemical reagent strips that have a component for examining LE, a marker for PMNs. When used with ascitic fluid from patients with cirrhosis or other liver diseases, the sensitivity ranged from approximately 50 to 100%, with wide confidence intervals. This indicates that many patients could be subjected to false negative tests. Nevertheless, as an alternative for use in the ambulatory setting or other acute care facilities that have limited laboratory resources, a colorimetric chemical reagent strip is an intriguing and innovative use of technology when applied in this way. It must be kept in mind that there are no data suggesting early treatment in the ED, or for the length of time it may take a regular laboratory to process ascitic fluid cell counts (in the order of 1–2 h), or how this test may improve outcomes or reduce mortality. However, the ease of use, widespread availability, and easy interpretation make this bedside point of care test promising and exciting. It must also be keep in mind that while there may be many commercially marketed urine dipsticks, the studies presented here only examined three different products. From a cost perspective, at approx 0.15 euros/strip for the Multistix and Nephur-test, it may well be cost-effective to pursue larger studies in order to better refine the test parameters on unselected patients with ascites.

References

1. Castellote, J., Lopez, C., Gornals, J., et al. (2003) Rapid diagnosis of spontaneous bacterial peritonitis by use of reagent strips. *Hepatology* **37**: 893–896.
2. Kim, D.Y., Kin, J.H., Chon, C.Y., et al. (2005) Usefulness of urine strip test in the rapid diagnosis of spontaneous bacterial peritonitis. *Liver International* **25**(6): 1197–1201.
3. Sapey, T., Kabissa, D., Fort, E., Laurin, C. and Mendler, M.H. (2005) Instant diagnosis of spontaneous bacterial peritonitis using leukocyte esterase reagent strips: Nephur-Test® vs. MultistixSG®. *Liver International* **25**(2): 343–348.

SECTION 5
Surgical and Abdominal Complaints

Chapter 28 Acute Nonspecific, Nontraumatic Abdominal Pain

> **Highlights**
>
> - The evaluation of undifferentiated abdominal pain may include an abdominal computed tomography (CT) scan when clinically indicated.
> - Compared to plain abdominal X-rays, noncontrast abdominal CT identifies intra-abdominal pathologies with higher sensitivity and specificity.

Background

Acute abdominal pain is one of the most common presenting complaints in the emergency department (ED). Recent developments in imaging techniques have dramatically changed the ED evaluation of abdominal pain. In contrast 15 to 20 years ago patients with abdominal pain traditionally received surgical consultations when it was decided whether to either take the patient to the operating room, admit and observe, or discharge the patient from the ED. Nowadays, because of the wide availability of imaging in the ED care often does not involve surgical consultation and frequently surgeons are involved after the results of laboratory tests and imaging studies are made available. Radiographic imaging modalities available in many EDs include plain abdominal radiography, CT (with or without intravenous and oral contrast), and ultrasound (US). Common blood tests such as white blood cell (WBC) counts are also often figured into the overall clinical evaluation. Almost 90% of the presentations with acute abdominal pain fall into one of eight diagnoses: appendicitis, bowel obstruction, cholecystitis, renal colic, peptic ulcer disease, pancreatitis, diverticular disease, and nonspecific abdominal pain.

With such a wide array of potential etiologies for abdominal pain, and the practical limitations that preclude performing every test and every imaging

Evidence-Based Emergency Care: Diagnostic Testing and Clinical Decision Rules. By J.M. Pines and W.W. Everett. Published 2008 by Blackwell Publishing, ISBN: 978-14051-5400-0.

procedure on every patient, the clinician must decided how to balance not imaging everyone and not missing serious causes for abdominal pain. In this chapter and the following four chapters, the discussion will focus on four of the most common clinical entities presenting as acute abdominal pain: bowel obstruction, and acute appendicitis, pancreatitis, and cholecystitis. To begin, the role of imaging in undifferentiated acute abdominal pain will be discussed.

Clinical question

"Which diagnostic imaging modality is most sensitive in diagnosing patients with undifferentiated acute abdominal pain?"

A retrospective descriptive study performed in 1994 examined a consecutive series of ED patients presenting with acute onset nontraumatic abdominal or flank pain who received both plain abdominal imaging (three view) and abdominal CT imaging (note that it was not specified in the study whether CTs were contrast or noncontrast).[1] Among 177 adult patients who received abdominal CT, 74 also received plain abdominal imaging. The gold standard diagnosis was determined from test results and the clinical outcomes recorded in the medical records. The results are shown in Table 28.1.

The authors found that the difference in imaging modality sensitivities and specificities were all statistically significant, with abdominal CT imaging

Table 28.1 Test parameters for plain film (PF) abdominal radiographs and abdominal computed tomography (CT) imaging (n = 74) from Nagurney *et al.*[1]

	PF			CT		
	Disease present (+)	Disease absent (−)	Total	Disease present (+)	Disease absent (−)	Total
Study abnormal (+)	25	4	29	53	1	54
Study normal (−)	33	12	45	5	15	20
Total	58	16	74	58	16	74
Sensitivity, % (95% CI)	43 (32–54)			91 (84–98)		
Specificity, % (95% CI)	75 (65–85)			94 (89–99)		
PPV, % (95% CI)	86 (78–94)			98 (95–100)		
NPV, % (95% CI)	27 (17–37)			75 (65–85)		
Diagnostic accuracy, % (95% CI)	50 (39–61)			92 (86–98)		

NPV, negative predictive value; PPV, positive predictive value.

performing uniformly better than plain abdominal radiography. They concluded that in patients with acute abdominal or flank pain in which a CT scan was likely to be obtained, there was minimal to no additional benefit from obtaining plain abdominal radiographs.

MacKersie *et al.* performed a prospective study of ED patients presenting with acute abdominal pain in which they compared noncontrast abdominal CT with three-view plain abdominal radiography.[2] They examined the test characteristics and diagnostic accuracy of the two imaging modalities compared to the final diagnosis made by surgical, pathological, and clinical follow-up at six months. Patients were enrolled if they had an onset of acute abdominal pain within the previous seven days. Patients were excluded if they were pregnant, intoxicated, lacked the mental capacity for decision making, or had vaginal bleeding, penile discharge, dysuria, or hematuria without flank pain. Interpreting radiologists were blinded to the study and to the clinical history of each patient.

Over a seven-month period 103 patients were enrolled, with 91 patients participating in both studies (Table 28.2). The final diagnoses included gastrointestinal diseases (n = 35) including acute appendicitis, cholecystitis, and pancreatitis, and diverticulitis, inflammatory bowel disease, hernias, and bowel obstructions; the remaining were diagnosed with either gynecological disease (n = 3), genitourinary disease (n = 8), metastatic disease (n = 4), or nonspecific abdominal pain (n = 41).

This study demonstrated that the noncontrast abdominal CT was better than plain films at revealing the cause of acute abdominal pain, including many of the concerning surgical or medically emergent/urgent causes. In many cases the CT led to the discovery of pathology that was not identified

Table 28.2 Diagnostic parameters comparing computed tomography (CT) and plain abdominal radiography (acute abdominal series, AAS) with the clinical outcome from MacKersie *et al.*[2]

	Outcome (+)	Outcome (−)	Total
CT (+)	48	2	50
CT (−)	2	39	41
Total	50	41	91
AAS (+)	15	5	20
AAS (−)	35	36	71
Total	50	41	91

AAS: sensitivity 30% (95% CI: 18–45), specificity 88% (95% CI: 74–96), accuracy 56%; CT: sensitivity 96% (95% CI: 86–100), specificity 95% (95% CI: 83–99), accuracy 96%.

using plain radiography. This study also demonstrated that noncontrast CT has sufficiently high sensitivity, specificity, and accuracy to makes it a useful imaging modality in the absence of any contrast, thus avoiding the risks of allergic reactions and contrast-induced nephropathy.

In another study, the diagnostic yields of both abdominal plain radiography and abdominal CT scanning were compared in a subset of patients presenting to an ED with undifferentiated acute abdominal pain.[3] Out of 1000 patients, only 120 received both plain abdominal imaging and abdominal CTs. This retrospective review of adult patients undergoing plain radiography (three view) in the first instance, followed by abdominal CT scanning with oral and intravenous contrast, examined the imaging performance parameters with respect to the outcome of final diagnosis, either at the time of ED or hospital discharge, for the following six diagnoses: bowel obstruction, urolithiasis, appendicitis, pyelonephritis, pancreatitis, and diverticulitis. Among this small sample there were 25 cases of urolithiasis, nine of diverticulitis, two of pyelonephritis, and three cases each for bowel obstruction, appendicitis, and pancreatitis. Plain abdominal radiography had sensitivities of 0% (95% CI: 0–84) for all but the bowel obstruction condition (sensitivity 33%; 95% CI: 25–42). The specificity for all of the diagnoses was 100% (95% CI: 96–100). The diagnostic accuracy of abdominal radiography ranged from 80 to 98%. Abdominal CT had sensitivities across all of the diagnoses ranging from 33 to 68% (95% CI: 25–76), with specificities ranging from 91 to 100% (95% CI: 85–100). The diagnostic accuracy of abdominal CT ranged from 86 to 98%. The authors concluded that plain abdominal radiography was insufficiently sensitive in the evaluation of acute nontraumatic abdominal pain.

Because of the difficulty in knowing exactly which laboratory tests, imaging studies, and history and physical examination findings are predictive of the need for acute medical or surgical interventions (defined as surgery or need for inpatient hospitalization) Gerhardt *et al.* examined 165 patients undergoing acute abdominal imaging and noncontrast helical CT scanning of the abdomen with nontraumatic, nonspecific abdominal pain.[4] Patients that were aged 18 years or older and that reported nontraumatic abdominal pain of up to seven days in duration were included. The authors found that when all of the data was aggregated, including the acute abdominal series results, the noncontrast abdominal CT was the most accurate clinical variable for an acute medical or surgical intervention. In a classification and regression tree analysis, the combination of history, physical examination, acute abdominal series imaging, and noncontrast abdominal CT imaging yielded the best test characteristics for predicting the need for medical or surgical intervention (sensitivity 92%, specificity 90%, positive predictive value 83%, negative predictive value 95%, accuracy 90%). Other models that did not include CT imaging had sensitivities and specificities that were felt to be unacceptably low. The authors concluded that from their derivation study guideline, that noncontrast abdominal CT was very useful and should be the imaging modality of choice when faced with nonspecific abdominal pain.

There are few good head-to-head comparative studies in the medical literature for different imaging modalities applicable to acute abdominal pain. Furthermore, studies performed using CT and US from as recently as 5–10 years ago may not be totally applicable today due to technological advances with each of these modalities. Many of these studies, including several of those reviewed here, suffer from a lack of uniform diagnostic gold standards, making broad comparisons between several similar studies difficult. Patients prospectively enrolled into the studies were often selected based upon a suspected diagnosis rather than an undifferentiated abdominal complaint, suggesting that some degree of selection bias was likely to be involved.

The use of oral and IV contrast dyes with abdominal CT scanning will continue to be a subject of debate. As CT is used more and more as the imaging modality of choice for acute abdominal pain, and specifically when bowel obstruction is being considered, there will continue to be an increase in the incidence of contrast nephropathy. Future studies are needed to compare contrast and noncontrast studies in order to minimize the iatrogenic effects of IV contrast. For patients with allergies or other contraindications for the use of IV contrast, the evidence supports the use of noncontrast CT as the diagnostic study of choice.

References

1. Nagurney, J.T., Brown, D.F.M., Novelline, R.A., Kim, J. and Fischer, R.H. (1999) Plain abdominal radiographs and abdominal CT scans for nontraumatic abdominal pain – added value? *American Journal of Emergency Medicine* **17**: 668–671.
2. MacKersie, A.B., Lane, M.J., Gerhardt, R.T., *et al.* (2005) Nontraumatic acute abdominal pain: unenhanced helical CT compared with three-view acute abdominal series. *Radiology* **237**: 114–122.
3. Ahn, S.H., Mayo-Smith, W.W., Murphy, B.L., Reinert, S.E. and Cronan, J.J. (2002) Acute nontraumatic abdominal pain in adult patients: abdominal radiography compared with CT evaluation. *Radiology* **225**: 159–164.
4. Gerhardt, R.T., Nelson, B.K., Keenan, S., Kernan, L., MacKersie, A. and Lane, M.S. (2005) Derivation of a clinical guideline for the assessment of nonspecific abdominal pain: the Guideline for Abdominal Pain in the ED Setting (GAPEDS) Phase 1 Study. *American Journal of Emergency Medicine* **25**: 709–717.

Background

Most patients with bowel obstruction will eventually seek acute medical evaluation. Bowel obstruction is a common cause of nontraumatic abdominal pain. The common causes of bowel obstruction include adhesions, hernias, malignancies, volvulus, inflammatory conditions, foreign bodies, gallstones, pancreatitis, intussusception, and closed-loop obstructions.

Clinical question one

"Which diagnostic imaging modality is most sensitive in diagnosing bowel obstruction?"

One of the first studies comparing abdominal CT with plain abdominal radiography (Fig. 29.1) in diagnosing small bowel obstruction was by Frager *et al.*[1] They studied a total of 85 patients on over 90 occasions in which each patient underwent both acute abdominal radiography (supine and erect images) and abdominal CT with intravenous (IV) and oral contrast. The gold standard for comparison was surgical outcome in 61 cases and clinical outcome in 29 cases. In cases where there was no obstruction (n = 24), plain films yielded a specificity of 88% (95% CI: 66–100) compared to CT,

---

Evidence-Based Emergency Care: Diagnostic Testing and Clinical Decision Rules. By J.M. Pines and W.W. Everett. Published 2008 by Blackwell Publishing, ISBN: 978-14051-5400-0.

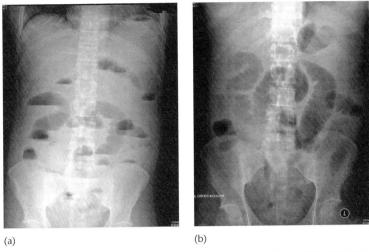

(a) (b)

Figure 29.1 Multiple air-fluid levels (a) and dilated loops of small bowel (b). (Courtesy of Anthony Dean, MD.)

which had a specificity of 83% (95% CI: 63–100). For cases of partial and complete small bowel obstruction (n = 20 and 46, respectively) the sensitivity of CT was 100% for both (95% CI: 78–100% and 92–100%, respectively), while plain films performed poorly with a sensitivity of 30% for partial obstruction (95% CI: 8–52) and 46% for complete obstruction (95% CI: 32–60). The authors concluded that the performance of abdominal CT was better than that of plain abdominal films for identifying partial and complete small bowel obstructions. CT provided additional information regarding the degree and location of the obstruction that helped to guide those cases requiring surgical intervention.

A small prospective study of 32 patients with acute abdominal pain was conducted in which the patients were evaluated with all of the following imaging modalities: plain abdominal radiographs (supine and erect view); abdominal CT with oral and IV contrast, and with and without rectal contrast; and abdominal ultrasound.[2] The study sought to compare the sensitivities, specificities, and accuracies of each imaging modality compared with the outcomes at surgery (n = 25) and clinical follow-up (n = 7). The interpreting radiologists were blinded to the findings from other imaging studies. All imaging occurred within a period of 6–36 h following presentation. The results are shown in Table 29.1 for the total of 30 bowel obstructions.

From this study it was concluded that CT yielded a significantly higher sensitivity than both ultrasound and plain radiography, and had 100%

Table 29.1 Test characteristics for diagnosing bowel obstruction among plain radiography, computed tomography (CT), and ultrasound (95% confidence intervals not provided in source study) from Suri et al.[2]

	Sensitivity, %	Specificity, %	Accuracy, %
Plain radiography	77	50	75
CT	93	100	94
Ultrasound	83	100	84

specificity. Furthermore, CT was able to identify the level and cause of the obstruction in 93 and 87% of cases, respectively, compared to ultrasound (70 and 23%, respectively) and plain radiography (60 and 7%, respectively). The causes of bowel obstruction were malignancy (n = 9), inflammation (n = 9), adhesions (n = 3), volvulus (n = 3), strictures (n = 3), intussusception (n = 2), and foreign body (n = 1).

When interpreting this data one must keep in mind the limitations of the study. For example, the time course over which the studies were performed may have impacted the ability to diagnose by a particular imaging modality. In addition the patient cohort was small. However, the performance of CT in this study is remarkable in terms of the high sensitivity shown, especially given the 100% specificity, and also in terms of its ability to accurately localize and diagnose the cause of the obstruction.

With few exceptions plain abdominal radiography has no role in the evaluation of suspected bowel obstruction. The exceptions include expected prolonged delay or absolute unavailability of CT imaging. Plain radiography is still used in other acute abdominal pain situations (foreign body ingestion, penetrating trauma, and suspected pneumoperitoneum), but its use is becoming rarer and therefore it is more difficult to learn about.

Newer imaging methods are being tested using MRI technology and the preliminary results look promising. In a prospective cross-sectional study of patients with clinical evidence of bowel obstruction, Beall et al. evaluated 44 patients that received rapid noncontrast MRI, IV contrast CT scanning, or both, and reported the following test characteristics: MRI sensitivity 95%, specificity 100%, accuracy 96%; and CT sensitivity 71%, specificity 71%, accuracy 71%.[3] In this study the total time taken for MRI, including patient set-up and image acquisition, was just under seven minutes. It is unclear why the CT had such low sensitivity and specificity in this small cohort compared to the previously cited studies. However, the possibility of a widespread use for MRI in the evaluation of acute abdominal pain remains a thought for the future.

References

1. Frager, D., Medwid, S.W., Baer, J.W., Mollinelli, B., Friedman, M. (1994) CT of small-bowel obstruction; value in establishing the diagnosis and determining the degree and cause. *American Journal of Roentgenology* **162**: 37–41.
2. Suri, S., Gupta, S., Sudhakar, P.J., Venkatataramu, N.K., Sood, B. and Wig, J.D. (1999) Comparative evaluation of plain films, ultrasound and CT in the diagnosis of intestinal obstruction. *Acta Radiologica* **40**: 422–428.
3. Beall, D.P., Fortman, B.J., Lawler, B.C. and Regan, F. (2002) Imaging bowel obstruction: a comparison between fast magnetic resonance imaging and helical computed tomography. *Clinical Radiology* **57**: 719–724.

Chapter 30 **Acute Pancreatitis**

Highlights

- Acute pancreatitis is commonly associated with alcohol use and gallstones and carries a mortality rate of approximately 1%.
- Serum lipase performs with excellent sensitivity and specificity compared to serum amylase in discriminating acute pancreatitis from other forms of acute abdominal pathology.

Background

Acute pancreatitis typically presents with abdominal pain, often in the epigastrium, with radiation through to the back. Excessive alcohol use and gallstones are the two most common risk factors for pancreatitis. Acute pancreatitis typically carries a mortality rate of approximately 1%, whereas 20% of cases constitute severe acute pancreatitis with mortality ranging from 10 to 25%. Two laboratory tests—serum amylase and lipase—are commonly obtained to help in the diagnosis of acute pancreatitis. Unfortunately, many of the studies examining the use of these tests utilize them as part of the diagnostic criteria for pancreatitis, thus artificially augmenting the sensitivity of the test.

Clinical question

"What is the role of serum amylase and lipase in the diagnosis of acute pancreatitis?"

Researchers in Germany studied amylase and lipase levels in a cohort of patients presenting to a university hospital for the evaluation of acute abdominal pain

Evidence-Based Emergency Care: Diagnostic Testing and Clinical Decision Rules. By J.M. Pines and W.W. Everett. Published 2008 by Blackwell Publishing, ISBN: 978-14051-5400-0.

suspected to be pancreatitis.[1] The gold standard used to classify patients as having pancreatitis was either contrast-enhanced computed tomography (CT) or abdominal ultrasound. Serum levels of amylase and lipase were taken at admission and within 48 h of the onset of symptoms. Of the total of 253 patients followed during the 10-month single hospital study, 32 (12.6%) were diagnosed by imaging with acute pancreatitis. For patients presenting within 48 h of symptom onset, an elevated lipase level had a sensitivity of 100% and a specificity of 84%, and an elevated amylase level had a sensitivity of 94% and a specificity of 88%. When diagnosis was based upon either of the initial tests being positive then the sensitivity was 100% and the specificity was 98%. An analysis of enzyme levels in the first serum draw compared to those in samples taken at days 2–3 and days 4–5 revealed that the sensitivity of the lipase assay fell to 59%, and that for the amylase assay fell to 35%. Receiver operating characteristic curve analysis showed the lipase assay to be slightly superior to the amylase assay, with 95% sensitivity achieved when lipase cutoff levels of two-fold above normal were used. From this study, the authors concluded that addition of serum amylase added only minimally to the diagnostic evaluation.

This study incorporated a definition of pancreatitis that did not include enzymatic parameters, and thus the enzyme performance parameters can be considered to be valid. The patients in this study may have been specifically selected because no data was provided regarding the total number of patients with abdominal pain who were not included, leaving clinicians to make suppositions about the study enrollment. Similarly, there was no mention of any other patients being identified with a final diagnosis of pancreatitis, thus cases may have been missed.

Researchers in New Zealand studied patients admitted to a single hospital over a three- to four-year period in which pancreatitis was a diagnostic consideration.[2] A total of 328 patients were consented and enrolled. The diagnosis of pancreatitis was based on a combination of factors, none of which included enzymatic determinations (operative-autopsy results, clinical features, and imaging results). Serum enzyme levels were determined on day one following presentation. A total of 51 patients were classified as having acute pancreatitis. The authors found that an elevated lipase level (above the diagnostic threshold) was 97% specific, but only 67% sensitive. This was significantly more discriminating compared to an elevated amylase level (specificity 97%, sensitivity 45%). The authors concluded that lipase was the preferred enzymatic study to perform in the initial presentation. The authors in this study focused on maximizing the specificity aspect of the diagnostic test as a way to avoid excessive false-positive results. The impact this has is to maximize the positive predictive value of a test.

Chapter 31 **Acute Appendicitis**

Highlights

- A white blood cell (WBC) count is insufficiently sensitive and specific, and lacks the predictive and discriminatory ability to diagnose acute appendicitis.
- Abdominal computed tomography (CT) is more sensitive than abdominal ultrasound (US) in diagnosing appendicitis and is the preferred imaging study in non-pregnant adults.
- Despite an increasing reliance on CT scans, the rates of missed and ruptured appendicitis have remained steady.

Background

Appendectomies are the most common emergency surgical procedures performed. Diagnosing acute appendicitis requires there to be a clinical suspicion after interviewing the patient, followed by a physical examination, and often diagnostic imaging. A surgical consultant is usually involved early on during a patient evaluation if there is a high clinical suspicion of appendicitis. In an effort to make a correct diagnosis, laboratory tests and imaging have increasingly been involved, with the hope being to reduce the number of missed or delayed diagnoses. However, the usefulness of specific laboratory tests and imaging studies in aiding the diagnosis has been questioned.

Clinical question one

"What is the role of the WBC count in the diagnosis of acute appendicitis?"
Two studies published in 2004 illustrate the lack of sufficient sensitivity and specificity for the total WBC count in diagnosing acute appendicitis. Cardall

Evidence-Based Emergency Care: Diagnostic Testing and Clinical Decision Rules. By J.M. Pines and W.W. Everett. Published 2008 by Blackwell Publishing, ISBN: 978-14051-5400-0.

Table 31.1 Test characteristics of white blood cell (WBC) counts in acute appendicitis from Cardall et al.[1]

	Appendicitis (+)	Appendicitis (−)	Total
WBC >10 000 cells/mm^3 (+)	66	89	155
WBC ≤10 000 cells/mm^3 (−)	21	98	119
Total	87	187	274
Sensitivity, % (95% CI)		76 (65–84)	
Specificity, % (95% CI)		52 (45–60)	
PPV, % (95% CI)		42 (35–51)	
NPV, % (95% CI)		82 (74–89)	
LR+ (95% CI)		1.59 (1.31–1.93)	
LR− (95% CI)		0.46 (0.31–0.67)	

LR, likelihood ratio; NPV, negative predictive value; PPV, positive predictive value.

et al. studied consecutive non-pregnant patients presenting to a single emergency department (ED) in which acute appendicitis was the working diagnosis after initial history and physical examination.[1] The diagnosis of appendicitis was based on surgical and histopathologic assessments. For patients who did not undergo an operation, follow-up was by telephone interviews two weeks later. A WBC count in excess of 10 000 cells/mm^3 was considered positive and was defined in this study *a priori*. A total of 293 patients had complete data for analysis, and the prevalence of acute appendicitis was found to be 31%. Table 31.1 shows the diagnostic test parameters. The area under the receiver operating characteristic (ROC) curve for the total WBC count was 0.72 (95% CI: 0.65–0.79), which is considered neither good [area under curve (AUC)>0.8] nor excellent (AUC>0.9). The authors concluded that the WBC count should not be relied upon to definitively rule in or rule out a working diagnosis of acute appendicitis because of its low sensitivity, low specificity and lack of discriminative power.

Anderson published a meta-analysis of laboratory values for diagnosing acute appendicitis.[2] In a review of the English, German, French, Italian, Spanish, Portuguese, and Scandinavian medical literature, the author found 24 articles that met the inclusion criteria, which consisted of studies with patients admitted to hospital for suspected appendicitis, studies including data permitting calculation of likelihood ratios and/or ROC curves, and studies including adult patients (pediatric-only studies were excluded). Diagnostic performance was determined using weighted pooled estimates of the area under the ROC curves and likelihood ratios for the diagnostic variables of interest. The results indicated that WBC counts had moderate discriminatory power, with a pooled area under the ROC curve of 0.77 (95% CI: 0.75–0.78).

Table 31.2 Likelihood ratios (LR) of elevated white blood cell (WBC) counts in diagnosing acute appendicitis in pooled studies from Anderson[2]

WBC (×10⁹/L)	LR+ (95% CI)	LR− (95% CI)
≥10	2.5 (2.1–3.0)	0.3 (0.2–0.4)
≥12	2.8 (2.0–3.8)	0.5 (0.4–0.6)
≥14	3.0 (2.5–3.5)	0.7 (0.6–0.9)
≥15	3.5 (1.6–7.8)	0.8 (0.7–1.0)

Higher WBC counts resulted in marginally better predictive capacity compared to lower WBC counts (Table 31.2).

This study demonstrated the lack of sufficient predictive and discriminatory ability of the total WBC count in diagnosing acute appendicitis. Indeed, the author performed calculations based on numerous permutations of inflammatory markers [WBC, C-reactive protein, proportion of polymorphonuclear cells (increased or decreased)] and found that only when two or more inflammatory markers were normal could there be sufficient confidence that appendicitis was unlikely.

Clinical question two

"Which diagnostic imaging modality is best for diagnosing acute appendicitis?"
The two common imaging studies used in the setting of suspected acute appendicitis are abdominal CT (Fig. 31.1) and US. Several studies have examined and compared the diagnostic yields and performances of these two modalities in settings in which both tests have been performed on all patients.

Pickuth *et al.* studied consecutive patients presenting with a suspicion of acute appendicitis over a six-month period.[3] All patients had noncontrast abdominal CT performed and abdominal US. The gold standard used for confirming the diagnosis was operative and pathologic findings for those undergoing surgery. Non-operative patients were followed after hospital discharge for six months. The prevalence of appendicitis was 78%. In the 27 patients without appendicitis, an alternative diagnosis was found in 15 (CT provided the alternative diagnosis in 14 cases; US provided an alternative diagnosis in nine cases). CT was accurate in 112/120 cases (93%), whereas US was accurate in 101/120 cases (84%; Table 31.3). The authors concluded that noncontrast abdominal CT yielded more accurate findings compared to US in patients with suspected acute appendicitis.

To further elucidate the diagnostic performance of abdominal CT versus focused right lower quadrant (RLQ) US, Wise *et al.* studied 100 consecutive

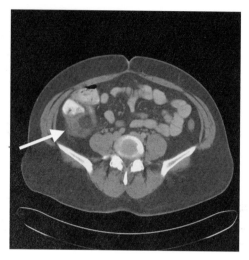

Figure 31.1 Computed tomography image showing tubular structure with surrounding fat stranding consistent with acute appendicitis (arrow).

Table 31.3 Diagnostic test performances of computed tomography (CT) and ultrasound (US) in acute appendicitis (n = 120) from Pickuth et al.[3]

	CT	US
Imaging study abnormal (+):		
Appendicitis (+)	88	81
Appendicitis (−)	3	7
Total	91	88
Imaging study normal (−):		
Appendicitis (+)	5	12
Appendicitis (−)	24	20
Total	29	32
Sensitivity, % (95% CI)	95 (89–98)	87 (79–93)
Specificity, % (95% CI)	89 (71–98)	74 (54–89)
PPV, % (95% CI)	97 (91–99)	92 (84–97)
NPV, % (95% CI)	83 (64–94)	63 (44–79)
LR+ (95% CI)	8.5 (2.9–24.8)	3.4 (1.8–6.4)
LR− (95% CI)	0.6 (0–0.1)	0.2 (0.1–0.3)

CT, computed tomography; LR, likelihood ratio; NPV, negative predictive value; PPV, positive predictive value; US, ultrasound.

patients presenting to an urban ED that were suspected of having acute appendicitis.[4] The subjects each underwent five diagnostic studies: (i) focused RLQ sonography; (ii) focused RLQ sonography following colonic contrast injection; (iii) focused abdominal CT of the appendiceal region following oral contrast; (iv) abdominopelvic CT following oral and intravenous (IV) contrast; and (v) focused abdominal CT of the cecal region following oral, IV, and colonic contrast injection. Imaging studies were interpreted blindly with regard to patients' clinical information, and CT and US studies were interpreted by different groups of radiologists. Outcomes were determined by surgical/pathology reports if an operation was performed, and by clinical follow-up for up to six-months if there was no surgery.

Overall, the prevalence of acute appendicitis was 24%. The authors reported that abdominal CT performed better than US diagnostically (CT sensitivity 96%, specificity 92%; US sensitivity 62%, specificity 71%; $P < 0.0001$). Furthermore, addition of IV or colonic contrast did not improve the performance of CT scanning.

The concern that prior studies that had examined selected patients in academic and university settings using specialized radiologists were not representative of general community practice was raised by a group of Dutch researchers.[5] The group went on to conduct a study of patients for whom there was a clinical suspicion of acute appendicitis, using both general and specialized radiologists. Of 339 patients with abdominal pain who were eligible for consent, 199 consented and underwent both noncontrast abdominal CT and RLQ US over a one-hour period. General radiologists (n = 10) and specialized radiologists (n = 2) blindly interpreted the studies. The outcomes were determined by surgical/pathology reports or by longitudinal follow-up, similar to other studies. Surgery was performed in 88% of the enrolled patients and the prevalence of acute appendicitis was 66%. The diagnostic performances of CT and US in this study were found to be statistically similar (Table 31.4).

A large systematic review of prospective studies examining the diagnostic accuracy of CT and US in diagnosing acute appendicitis was conducted in 2004.[6] Studies spanning 15 years (1988–2003) that utilized either abdominal CT or US, that enrolled patients that were above 13 years of age, and that incorporated surgical or clinical follow-up were included. The authors reported that, overall, CT performed better than US (Table 31.5).

The main limitation identified by the authors of all of the studies mentioned above was the use of different reference standards for patients with positive or negative tests. The studies cited used combinations of surgical and pathologic assessments and clinical follow-up, introducing bias when a uniform outcome standard was not utilized. Similarly, most studies included

Table 31.4 Diagnostic parameters comparing computed tomography (CT) and ultrasound (US) from Poortman et al.[5]

	Appendicitis (+)	Appendicitis (−)	Total
CT (+)	100	11	111
CT (−)	32	56	88
Total	132	67	199
US (+)	104	15	119
US (−)	28	52	80
Total	132	67	199

CT: sensitivity 76% (95% CI 68–83), specificity 83% (95% CI 73–92), accuracy 78%; US: sensitivity 79% (95% CI 71–85), specificity 78% (95% CI 66–87), accuracy 78%.

Table 31.5 Summary performance of computed tomography (CT) and ultrasound (US) in diagnosing appendicitis from Terasawa et al.[6]

	Sensitivity, % (95% CI)	Specificity, % (95% CI)	LR+ (95% CI)	LR− (95% CI)
CT	94 (91–95)	95 (93–96)	13.3 (9.9–17.9)	0.09 (0.07–0.12)
US	86 (83–88)	81 (78–84)	5.8 (3.5–9.5)	0.19 (0.13–0.27)

LR, likelihood ratio.

in this assessment reported the severity of disease, which is a form of spectrum bias.

Finally, Flum *et al.* performed a population-based analysis of misdiagnosis rates among patients undergoing appendectomies.[7] They examined the hypothesis that with increasing use of imaging among at-risk populations, there would be an expected decrease in the rate of missed appendicitis. However, an evaluation of population-based data from Washington State found that there was no statistical change in the misdiagnosis rate over a 12-year period (1987–1998). The rates of ruptured and misdiagnosed appendicitis were stable at approximately 2.6 and 1.6 cases per 10 000 person-years, respectively.

Taking into account these limitations, we believe that several take-home points emerge from the data. First, the reliance on the total WBC count in acute appendicitis is overstated and overutilized in clinical practice. In an era of cost containment where test selection is being followed closely, continued use of a blood test such as the WBC count to completely rule out a final diagnosis can no longer be supported.

For the diagnosis of bowel obstruction and acute appendicitis CT is the superior imaging modality compared with the other widely available imaging modalities (plain abdominal radiography and US). The use of abdominal CT imaging has several advantages over the other methods. In addition to making the diagnosis, the level of the obstruction and the cause of the obstruction can be better delineated. Alternative causes for the abdominal pain, such as a leaking aortic aneurysm for example, can also be diagnosed. The principal criticism for the widespread use of CT as the first imaging modality relates to indiscriminate radiation exposure compared with limited plain abdominal imaging, which is associated with only minimal radiation exposure, or US/magnetic resonance imaging (MRI) which has no ionizing radiation exposure. The use of US in the evaluation of intestinal pathology is limited due to the presence of bowel gas and obesity, and due to the fact that it is highly user dependent. With the exception of selected populations, specifically pediatric patients (not discussed here), US is frequently insufficient or non-diagnostic and thus a follow-up study is needed.

References

1. Cardall, T., Glasser, J. and Guss, D.A. (2004) Clinical value of the total white blood cell count and temperature in the evaluation of patients with suspected appendicitis. *Academic Emergency Medicine* **11**: 1021–1027.
2. Anderson, R.E.B. (2004) Meta-analysis of the clinical and laboratory diagnosis of appendicitis. *British Journal of Surgery* **91**: 28–37.
3. Pickuth, D., Heywang-Kobrunner, S.H. and Spielmann, R.P. (2000) Suspected acute appendicitis: is ultrasound or computed tomography the preferred imaging technique? *European Journal of Surgery* **166**: 315–319.
4. Wise, S.W., Labuski, M.R., Kasales, C.J., *et al.* (2001) Comparative assessment of CT and sonographic techniques for appendiceal imaging. *American Journal of Roentgenology* **176**: 933–941.
5. Poortman, P., Lohle, P.N.M., Schoemaker, C.M.C., *et al.* (2003) Comparison of CT and sonography in the diagnosis of acute appendicitis: a blinded prospective study. *American Journal of Roentgenology* **181**: 1355–1359.
6. Terasawa, T., Blackmore, C.C., Bent, S. and Kohlwes, R.J. (2004) Systematic review: computed tomography and ultrasonography to detect acute appendicitis in adults and adolescents. *Annals of Internal Medicine* **141**: 537–546.
7. Flum, D.R., Morris, A., Koepsell, T. and Dellinger, E.P. (2001) Has misdiagnosis of appendicitis decreased over time? *Journal of the American Medical Association* **286**: 1748–1753.

Chapter 32 **Acute Cholecystitis**

Highlights

- History, physical examination findings, and laboratory values are not sensitive predictors of acute cholecystitis.
- Gallbladder imaging can be performed with ultrasound (US), computed tomography (CT), and hepatobiliary scintigraphy (HIDA); however, each modality carries different advantages and disadvantages.

Background

Acute cholecystitis is a common concern among patients presenting for the evaluation of acute abdominal pain, accounting for approximately 5–9% of such admissions. Similar to the previously discussed concerns with diagnosing bowel obstruction (Chapter 29), acute pancreatitis (Chapter 30), and acute appendicitis (Chapter 31), the diagnosis entails a combination of historical and physical examination features coupled with appropriate imaging studies.

Clinical question

"Which diagnostic imaging test is recommended for diagnosing acute cholecystitis?"

Radiologists at the University of Pennsylvania compared abdominal CT with oral and intravenous (IV) contrast to US for the diagnosis of acute biliary disease (Figs 32.1 and 32.2) in a retrospective cohort of patients that underwent both imaging studies.[1] Patients were included if they had right upper quadrant (RUQ) pain and both RUQ US and abdominal CT imaging studies were performed within 48 h of each other. Patients with prior cholecystectomy

---

Evidence-Based Emergency Care: Diagnostic Testing and Clinical Decision Rules. By J.M. Pines and W.W. Everett. Published 2008 by Blackwell Publishing, ISBN: 978-14051-5400-0.

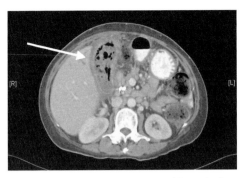

Figure 32.1 Oral contrast CT showing air-filled gallbladder and inflammation surrounding the gallbladder wall consistent with emphysematous cholecystitis (arrow).

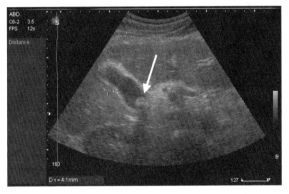

Figure 32.2 Transabdominal ultrasound showing thickened gallbladder wall with a stone in the gallbladder (arrow). The calipers demonstrate that the gallbladder wall measures 4.1 mm. (Courtesy of Anthony Dean, MD)

were excluded. CT and US studies were blindly interpreted by separate radiologists and a final diagnosis of acute cholecystitis was determined by surgical and pathology reports, and autopsy findings. The objective in this study was to determine which the most appropriate imaging modality to employ first was. For our purposes, the study provides the opportunity to examine the performances of the two imaging modalities for the diagnosis of acute biliary disease (shown in Table 32.1). The study identified 123 patients, of which 117 were suspected of having acute biliary disease. A final diagnosis of acute cholecystitis was made in 18 patients (incidence 15%) in this study group.

The authors concluded among other things that RUQ US was the preferred first study when considering a diagnosis of acute biliary disease, with a signi-

Table 32.1 Computed tomography (CT) and ultrasound (US) performances for the diagnosis of acute biliary disease from Harvey and Miller[1]

	Acute biliary disease (+)	Acute biliary disease (−)	Total
CT (+)	7	7	14
CT (indeterminate or −)	11	92	103
Total	18	99	117
US (+)	15	5	20
US (indeterminate or −)	3	94	97
Total	18	99	117

CT: sensitivity 39% (95% CI: 17–64), specificity 93% (95% CI: 86–97), accuracy 85%; US: sensitivity 83% (95% CI: 59–96), specificity 95% (95% CI: 89–98), accuracy 93%.

ficantly better sensitivity and marginally higher specificity compared to abdominal CT. It was specifically noted, however, that if other factors were under diagnostic consideration in the differential diagnosis then CT should still be considered.

HIDA has long been considered the gold standard for diagnosing acute cholecystitis. In a retrospective analysis of patients presenting to a single center with suspected acute cholecystitis that had both US and HIDA ordered simultaneously, the performance characteristics of the two tests were compared.[2] It was standard practice in the study hospital for both studies to be ordered together when this diagnosis was being considered. Consecutive patients were included; patients were excluded if a test was ordered after the first test had been completed in an effort to minimize differential test ordering bias. The final diagnosis was determined using surgical, pathology, and autopsy reports, or via a clinical diagnosis for those who did not die or undergo surgery. A total of 107 patients were examined and 32 (30%) had a final diagnosis of acute cholecystitis. Using data from this study, the performance characteristics of the two tests are shown in Table 32.2.

The authors concluded that HIDA was superior in diagnosing acute cholecystitis. They suggested that the costs of each of these studies at the time were sufficiently similar that the decision should be based on availability and diagnostic performance.

Finally, to highlight the importance of selecting the correct imaging study, Trowbridge and colleagues performed a comprehensive review of studies examining the ability of physical examination, patient history, or laboratory tests to diagnose acute cholecystitis.[3] They found no historic or clinical factors that could sufficiently rule in or rule out acute cholecystitis (LR+ ≤2.8; LR− <0.4), indirectly supporting the notion that imaging is the cornerstone of diagnosis.

Table 32.2 Test characteristics of hepatobiliary scintigraphy (HIDA) and ultrasound (US) for cholecystitis from Chatziioannou et al.[2]

	Acute biliary disease (+)	Acute biliary disease (−)	Total
HIDA (+)	28	5	33
HIDA (−)	4	70	74
Total	32	75	107
US (+)	16	9	25
US (indeterminate or −)	16	66	82
Total	32	75	107

HIDA: sensitivity 88% (95% CI: 71–97), specificity 93% (95% CI: 85–98), accuracy 92%; US: sensitivity 50% (95% CI: 32–68), specificity 88% (95% CI: 78–94), accuracy 77%.

Comments

While CT is regarded as the study of choice, and this is supported by data for many abdominal conditions, US is very useful and is a reasonable diagnostic choice in acute biliary diseases. HIDA has been shown to have superior test parameters, but the lack of widespread availability and access during off-hours are the main factors limiting its use.

References

1. Harvey, R.T. and Miller, W.T., Jr. (1999) Acute biliary diseases: initial CT and follow-up US versus initial US and follow-up CT. *Radiology* **13**: 831–836.
2. Chatziioannou, S.N., Moore, W.H., Ford, P.V. and Dhekne, R.D. (2000) Hepatobiliary scintigraphy is superior to abdominal ultrasonography in suspected acute cholecystitis. *Surgery* **127**: 609–613.
3. Trowbridge, R.L., Rutkowski, N.K. and Shojania, K.G. (2003) Does this patient have acute cholecystitis? *Journal of the American Medical Association* **289**(1): 80–86.

SECTION 6
Urology

Chapter 33 **Kidney Stones**

Highlights

- Kidney stones should be considered in patients presenting with acute flank pain, hematuria, groin pain, and/or vomiting.
- Noncontrast computed tomography (CT) imaging in patients with suspected kidney stones improves the diagnostic accuracy and can provide important information about other unsuspected conditions, some of which may require emergency treatment.

Background

Kidney stones affect up to 5% of the population. People frequently seek emergency care for pain associated with kidney stones because it is frequently severe and refractory to over-the-counter medications. Clinical features of symptomatic kidney stones include acute flank pain radiating to the groin, nausea, vomiting, and microscopic hematuria. The standard for the diagnosis of kidney stones is noncontrast spiral CT scanning (Fig. 33.1). Noncontrast CT has become the standard because it gives a considerable amount of information including the following: (i) whether the symptoms are actually due to kidney stones; (ii) whether the stones are obstructing; and (iii) an estimate of the stone burden if the scan is positive (Fig. 33.2). An estimate of stone burden may be helpful for physicians in managing an individual patient's kidney stones after their emergency department (ED) visit. When a patient develops kidney stones, in almost 50% of cases a second stone will form within 5–7 years.

Evidence-Based Emergency Care: Diagnostic Testing and Clinical Decision Rules. By J.M. Pines and W.W. Everett. Published 2008 by Blackwell Publishing, ISBN: 978-14051-5400-0.

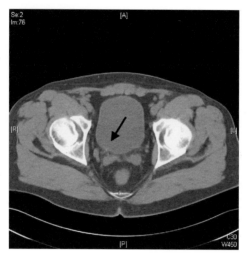

Figure 33.1 Noncontrast computed tomography scan showing 1–2 mm calculus at the right ureterovescicular junction (arrow).

Clinical question one

"How does unenhanced CT compare to other diagnostic tests for kidney stones, including intravenous (IV) urography and ultrasound (US)?"

A recent randomized trial was performed comparing CT to IV urography for patients with suspected nephrolithasis.[1] The authors enrolled 122 patients with acute flank pain and suspected kidney stones. A total of 59 were randomized to CT and 63 to IV urography, and the radiographic studies were independently interpreted by four radiologists. Of the 63 patients receiving IV urography, mild to moderate adverse reactions from contrast material were seen in three (5%). The mean radiation dose was 3.3 mSv for urography and 6.5 mSv for CT scans. The sensitivity and specificity for CT were 94.1 and 94.2%, respectively. For urography, sensitivity and specificity were poorer at 85.2 and 90.4%, respectively.

Another recent study investigated the sensitivity of diagnostic US compared to CT for detecting kidney stones in 46 patients with acute flank pain.[2] CT scanning detected 22 of 23 ureteral calculi (sensitivity 96%) and US detected 14 of 23 ureteral calculi (sensitivity 61%). The specificity for each technique was 100%. When modalities were compared for the detection of any clinically relevant abnormality, the sensitivities of US and CT were 92 and 100%, respectively.

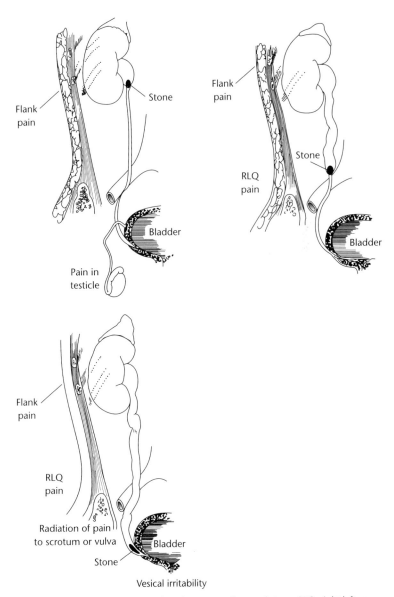

Figure 33.2 Radiation of pain with various types of ureteral stone. RLQ, right left quadrant. (Source: Tanagho and McAninch, *Smith's General Urology* 16th Edition © 2004. Reproduced with permission of The McGraw-Hill Companies.)

Clinical question two

"Is it important to use noncontrast CT to diagnose kidney stones on the first visit for presumed ureteral colic?"

A prospective observational study assessed the impact of helical CT in 132 patients presenting with their first episode of suspected nephrolithiasis.[3] Patients with a known history of kidney stones were excluded. Prior to the CT, emergency physicians completed questionnaires detailing the diagnostic certainty of nephrolithiasis and anticipated disposition. The primary study outcome was physician diagnostic certainty compared to CT results. The secondary outcome measure was an alternate diagnosis. There were four categories grouped in terms of pre-CT diagnostic certainty: 0–49%, 50–74%, 75–90%, and 90–100%. These categories were associated with a diagnosis of urinary calculi in 28.6, 45.7, 74.2, and 80.5% of patients, respectively. CT scans revealed an alternative diagnosis in 40 cases (33%). Of these, 19 had another significant pathology the majority of which were previously unrecognized cancers; some were less significant, such as adrenal adenomas. Before CT scanning, physicians planned to discharge 115 patients and admit six patients. The authors concluded that patients presenting with a first episode of clinically suspected nephrolithiasis should undergo a CT scan because it enhances and hence improves diagnostic accuracy and identifies clinically significant alternative diagnoses.

Another more recent study examined the incidence and clinical relevance of alternate diagnoses in a large series of 1500 patients with acute flank pain and suspected urinary calculi that received a CT scan.[4] In this study patients with a history of urinary tract calculi were not excluded. Alternate findings on CT scans were classified in terms of whether they required immediate or delayed treatment, or were of little or no clinical importance. They found that 69% in this series had urinary tract calculi. This included 30% with nephrolithiasis, 36% with ureterolithiasis, and 34% with both conditions. Of all patients 1064 (71%) had other or additional CT findings, 207 (14%) had non-kidney stone related CT findings requiring immediate or deferred treatment, 464 (31%) had pathological conditions of little clinical importance, and 393 (26%) had pathological conditions of no clinical relevance. The authors concluded that in patients with acute flank pain, CT allows the accurate diagnosis of urinary stone disease and can provide further important information leading to emergency treatment in a substantial number of patients.

Comment

It appears that the noncontrast CT scan is the diagnostic test of choice in patients with suspected nephrolithasis. CT is considerably more accurate than other testing modalities, such as IV urography or diagnostic ultrasound. For patients with a first episode of suspected nephrolithasis, CT scanning should be used as it can confirm the presence of kidney stones and has the potential to find other clinically significant pathologies in a considerable number of cases.

References

1. Pfister, S.A., Deckart, A., Laschke, S., *et al.* (2003) Unenhanced helical computed tomography vs intravenous urography in patients with acute flank pain: accuracy and economic impact in a randomized prospective trial. *European Radiology* **13**: 2513–2520.
2. Sheafor, D.H., Hertzberg, B.S., Freed, K.S., *et al.* (2000) Nonenhanced helical CT and US in the emergency evaluation of patients with renal colic: prospective comparison. *Radiology* **217**: 792–797.
3. Ha, M. and MacDonald, R.D. (2004) Impact of CT scan in patients with first episode of suspected nephrolithasis. *Journal of Emergency Medicine* **27**: 225–231.
4. Hoppe, H., Studer, R., Kessler, T.M., *et al.* (2006) Alternate or additional findings to stone disease on unenhanced computerized tomography for acute flank pain can impact management. *Journal of Urology* **175**: 1725–1730.

Chapter 34 **Testicular Torsion**

Highlights

- Acute testicular torsion is a urological emergency and should be considered in males presenting with testicular or scrotal pain.
- Testicular ultrasound (US) is widely available, highly accurate, and is considered the study of choice.
- High-resolution ultrasonography (HRUS), which directly images the spermatic cord, detects testicular torsion with high sensitivity and specificity; however, it may not be widely available.

Background

The patient with testicular pain presents a diagnostic challenge for emergency physicians. There are multiple causes for testicular pain including infectious and inflammatory reasons, neoplasms, hernias, acute trauma, and torsion. For those under the age of 25, testicular torsion occurs annually in approximately 1 in 4000 males. Torsion should be considered in the differential diagnosis for every male presenting with testicular or scrotal pain, but it is predominately a condition of the young and very young. Commonly, a twisting of the spermatic cord compromises the blood flow and causes acute pain. Obstruction of venous flow is the first finding of testicular torsion followed by arterial. The end result is testicular ischemia.

Testicular torsion is considered a urological emergency. Ruling out testicular torsion is important and time-sensitive because delays in diagnosis and therapy can result in problems with fertility, organ loss, and a poor cosmetic outcome. Viability and salvageability of the torsed testicle decreases as the time from the onset of symptoms (e.g. pain) increases, with approximately

---

Evidence-Based Emergency Care: Diagnostic Testing and Clinical Decision Rules. By J.M. Pines and W.W. Everett. Published 2008 by Blackwell Publishing, ISBN: 978-14051-5400-0.

90% salvageability if detorsion is performed less than 6 h after onset, almost 50% viability after 12 h, and close to 10% after 24 h. In the emergency department (ED), scintigraphy or US have become standard practice for diagnosing testicular torsion. The limited widespread availability of nuclear imaging has further restricted the use of testicular scintigraphy, resulting in testicular US being the usual imaging study ordered for this uncommon condition.

Clinical question

"What are the sensitivities and specificities of testicular scintigraphy compared to testicular US for the diagnosis of testicular torsion?"
Several studies have compared testicular scintigraphy with testicular US. A 1990 study prospectively evaluated 28 males with acute scrotal pain ranging in age from one day old to 41 years.[1] Patients with classic testicular torsion symptoms were taken directly to the operating room and were therefore excluded from the study. All remaining patients underwent testicular scintigraphy using technetium-99m pertechnetate as well as color Doppler US using a 7.5-MHz linear probe. Studies were interpreted by the physician performing the study who had full knowledge of the clinical histories. Seven testicular torsion cases were identified at surgery (25%) and no cases were missed at follow-up. The performances of each diagnostic modality are shown in Table 34.1.

Not all patients underwent surgical exploration and therefore a hybridized gold standard of a combination of clinical follow-up and surgical outcome was used. The authors noted that color Doppler US permitted differentiation of other causes of acute scrotal pain, notably epididymitis and orchitis.

Table 34.1 Test performances of testicular color Doppler ultrasound (US) and testicular scintigraphy for the diagnosis of acute testicular torsion from Middleton *et al.*[1]

	Testicular torsion (+)	Testicular torsion (−)	Total
Color Doppler US (+)	7	0	7
Color Doppler US (−)	0	21	21
Total	7	21	28
Testicular scintigraphy (+)	6	0	6
Testicular scintigraphy (−)	1	21	22
Total	7	21	28

Color Doppler US: sensitivity 100% (95% CI: 59–100), specificity 100% (95% CI: 84–100); testicular scintigraphy: sensitivity 86% (95% CI: 42–100), specificity 100% (95% CI: 84–100).

However, the small sample size precluded the recommendation of color Doppler US as the preferred modality.

A retrospective pediatric study of 41 boys with acute scrotal pain and equivocal physical examinations from 1990 to 1996 compared the performance of color Doppler US with testicular scintigraphy for the diagnosis of testicular torsion.[2] Patients were followed through surgery or clinically until the symptoms were resolved. A total of 11 cases (27%) of torsion occurred. Several studies were interpreted as being non-diagnostic. The authors presented two sets of performance tables, one that treated indeterminate studies as being positive for torsion (see Table 34.2) and another that treated indeterminate cases as being negative for torsion (see Table 34.3). The data presented

Table 34.2 Performance of color Doppler ultrasound (US) and testicular scintigraphy for diagnosing testicular torsion when the indeterminate studies were considered positive for torsion from Paltiel et al.[2]

	Torsion (+)	Torsion (−)	Total
Color Doppler US (+)	11	7	18
Color Doppler US (−)	0	23	23
Total	11	30	41
Testicular scintigraphy (+)	11	1	12
Testicular scintigraphy (−)	0	29	29
Total	11	30	41

Color Doppler US: sensitivity 100% (95% CI: 72–100), specificity 77% (95% CI: 58–90); testicular scintigraphy: sensitivity 100% (95% CI: 72–100), specificity 97% (95% CI: 83–100).

Table 34.3 Performance of color Doppler ultrasound (US) and testicular scintigraphy for diagnosing testicular torsion when the indeterminate studies were considered negative for torsion from Paltiel et al.[2]

	Torsion (+)	Torsion (−)	Total
Color Doppler US (+)	9	1	10
Color Doppler US (−)	2	29	31
Total	11	30	41
Testicular scintigraphy (+)	10	0	10
Testicular scintigraphy (−)	1	30	31
Total	11	30	41

Color Doppler US: sensitivity 82% (95% CI: 48–98), specificity 97% (95% CI: 83–100); testicular scintigraphy: sensitivity 91% (95% CI: 59–100), specificity 100% (95% CI: 88–100).

in this way is a sensitivity analysis of sorts, showing the effect that indeterminate cases have on the diagnostic performance of the tests.

The weaknesses of the retrospective design of the previous study prompted a prospective analysis of children comparing the same diagnostic tests.[3] Forty-six children with acute scrotal pain that received both testicular scintigraphy and US were enrolled. The final diagnosis was determined surgically in 16 cases and by following the clinical resolution in 30 boys. A total of 14 cases of torsion were diagnosed in this study (34%); 12 had testicular torsion proven at surgery, one case was detected based on an antecedent torsion and testicular atrophy, and one case of late testicular torsion was detected at follow-up.

The correct diagnosis of torsion was made by US in 11 out of 14 cases (sensitivity 79%, 95% CI: 49–95) and the correct diagnosis of non-surgical conditions was made in 31 out of 32 cases (specificity 97%, 95% CI: 84–100). The positive predictive value (PPV) and negative predictive value (NPV) for US were 92% (95%CI: 62–100) and 91% (95% CI: 76–98), respectively. Using US yielded a diagnostic accuracy of 91%. The correct diagnosis of torsion was made by scintigraphy in 11 of 14 cases (sensitivity 79%, 95% CI: 49–96) and the correct diagnosis of non-surgical conditions was made in 29 of 32 cases (specificity 91%, 95% CI: 75–98). The PPV and NPV for scintigraphy were 79% (95% CI: 49–95) and 91% (95% CI: 75–98), respectively. Scintigraphy resulted in a diagnostic accuracy of 87%.

The lack of a true gold standard imaging test is demonstrated by the false negatives seen in this study. The authors noted that one of the difficulties in diagnosing normal blood flow, not to mention the detection of abnormal or absent blood flow, was the small size of the prepubescent testicles.

From 1999 to 2005 European researchers studying the diagnosis of testicular torsion examined 61 infants and children ranging in age from one day old to 17 years presenting with acute scrotal pain, swelling, and redness.[4] All patients underwent color Doppler US. Fifteen cases of torsion were detected (25%)—14 by the absence of venous pulsation and one by the absence of arterial pulsations—and all were surgically confirmed with no missed cases. Forty-six non-torsion cases were also diagnosed correctly. Table 34.4 shows the performance of color Doppler US for the diagnosis of testicular torsion.

These authors also performed a retrospective analysis of 75 acute scrotum cases from 1985 to 1994, before the start of the study described above. All cases of suspected testicular torsion were explored surgically. Only 25 of the 75 cases (33%) were confirmed as torsion. These data were used as supporting evidence to demonstrate that the use of testicular US reduced the incidence of unnecessary surgical explorations.

Table 34.4 Performance of color Doppler ultrasound (US) for diagnosing acute testicular torsion in pediatric patients from Gunther *et al.*[4]

	Torsion (+)	Torsion (−)	Total
Color Doppler US (+)	15	0	15
Color Doppler US (−)	0	46	46
Total	15	46	61
Sensitivity, % (95% CI)		100 (78–100)	
Specificity, % (95% CI)		100 (92–100)	
PPV, % (95% CI)		100 (78–100)	
NPV, % (95% CI)		100 (92–100)	

NPV, negative predictive value; PPV, positive predictive value.

The most recent modality to be tested for the diagnosis of testicular torsion is HRUS. This technique images the spermatic cord to enable twisting of the cord to be visualized directly. In a European multicenter study, children with acute scrotal pain were imaged using both color Doppler US and HRUS.[5] The study enrolled 919 patients from 1992 to 2005 (age range one day old to 18 years). Spermatic cord torsion was diagnosed in 208 patients (23%). Using color Doppler US 158 of the 208 cases were detected (sensitivity 76%, 95% CI: 70–82), whereas HRUS detected 199 of the 208 cases (sensitivity 96%, 95% CI: 92–98). Calculation of the specificity of US could not be calculated from the data presented. The specificity of HRUS was 99% (95% CI: 98–100) with 705 of 711 cases revealing a linear (normal) spermatic cord. The PPV and NPV for HRUS were 97% (95% CI: 94–99) and 99% (95% CI: 98–99), respectively.

Comments

The current practice environment for evaluation of the acute scrotum endorses either prompt surgical evaluation by a skilled urologist or, more commonly, a diagnostic imaging study to aid in ruling out testicular torsion. Patients presenting with 'classic' findings of acute onset of pain, a high riding testicle, or other features that make the likelihood of acute torsion moderate or high, should not require a diagnostic test but rather should go directly to the operating room for surgical exploration. It is cases in which the history, physical findings, or both are equivocal that should prompt the use of a diagnostic imaging study.

The array of studies presented here demonstrate several key findings. First, regardless of the type of imaging study, none have been shown to be perfectly sensitive or specific in any large study. Technological advances and newer uses for existing diagnostic equipment continue to increase diagnostic thresholds, and these have to be considered when conducting a review of the literature. Cases in which the clinical suspicion is great enough to warrant ordering a study and cases in which the study results are indeterminate or poor quality warrant a urological consultation. Second, clinicians should consider the experience of the diagnostician interpreting the study. Finally, while this discussion has focused on using the imaging studies to rule out testicular torsion, US has the added advantage of providing an alternative diagnosis for conditions such as epididymitis, orchitis, and torsion of the testicular appendages.

The availability of US is greater than that of nuclear scintigraphy, making it the study of choice. Clinicians with no access to either of these modalities, or with no surgical backup available to perform the procedure, should arrange to transfer the patient to a medical facility that is capable of performing both the diagnostic study and the surgical procedure, as required for a positive diagnosis.

References

1. Middleton, W.D., Siegel, B.A., Melson, G.L., Yates, C.K. and Andriole, G.L. (1990) Acute scrotal disorders: prospective comparison of color Doppler US and testicular scintigraphy. *Radiology* **177**(1): 177–181.
2. Paltiel, H.J., Connolly, L.P., Atala, A., Paltiel, A.D., Zurakowski, D. and Treves, S.T. (1998) Acute scrotal symptoms in boys with an indeterminate clinical presentation: comparison of color Doppler sonography and scintigraphy. *Radiology* **207**(1): 223–231.
3. Blask, A.R.N., Bulas, D., Shalaby-Rana, E., Rushton, G., Shao, C. and Majd, M. (2002) Color Doppler sonography and scintigraphy of the testis: a prospective, comparative analysis in children with acute scrotal pain. *Pediatric Emergency Care* **18**(2): 67–71.
4. Gunther, P., Schenk, J.P., Wunsch, R., *et al.* (2006) Acute testicular torsion in children: the role of sonography in the diagnostic workup. *European Radiology* **16**: 2527–2532.
5. Kalfa, N., Veyrac, C., Lopez, M., *et al.* (2007) Multicenter assessment of ultrasound of the spermatic cord in children with acute scrotum. *Journal of Urology* **177**: 297–301.

SECTION 7
Neurology

Chapter 35 **Subarachnoid Hemorrhage**

Highlights

- Noncontrast head computed tomography (CT) is the best initial imaging study for diagnosing acute subarachnoid hemorrhage in the emergency department (ED).
- Newer generation CT scanners have better diagnostic accuracy but may not be available in all EDs.
- Lumbar puncture (LP) should be considered in patients with negative head CTs who are still suspected of having the condition, particularly when there is a high pre-test probability.
- There are no clinical decision rules or prediction rules regarding who should undergo testing for subarachnoid hemorrhage or what constitutes a positive LP.

Background

There are about five million ED visits per year for headache. Of those, between 1 and 4% have nontraumatic subarachnoid hemorrhage (SAH). Nontraumatic SAH is frequently caused by a ruptured cerebral aneurysm or an arteriovenous malformation. Extravasation of blood into the subarachnoid space negatively affects local and global brain function. Depending upon the size of the bleed, SAH can be fatal immediately; however, in cases of smaller bleeds, patients can present with severe headaches. SAH is a challenge for emergency providers because it can present in subtle ways and is associated with considerable morbidity and mortality. SAH is typically diagnosed on nonconstrast head CT. However, head CT is not 100% sensitive for SAH and is particularly insensitive for diagnosing small intracranial bleeds or

---

Evidence-Based Emergency Care: Diagnostic Testing and Clinical Decision Rules. By J.M. Pines and W.W. Everett. Published 2008 by Blackwell Publishing, ISBN: 978-14051-5400-0.

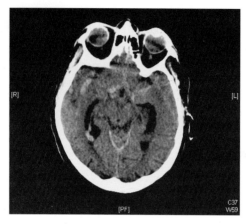

Figure 35.1 Noncontrast head computed tomography showing a subarachnoid bleed.

bleeding that is temporally distant from the ED presentation of headache. Because the greatest risk for rebleeding occurs within a month of the first sentient bleed, a timely and accurate diagnosis is vital for managing SAH and minimizing complications. Currently the gold standard for diagnosing SAH is LP, which will demonstrate either a high red blood cell count in the cerebrospinal fluid (CSF) or xanthochromia (a yellowing of the CSF secondary to breakdown products of red blood cells). LP and CSF analysis can also reveal other information that can be useful to clinicians, such as an elevation in intracranial pressure or the presence of infection.

There is no validated decision rule for predicting which patients require testing for SAH in the ED.[1] A recent decision rule was derived for the detection of SAH in ED patients with acute headache in six centers, which listed four criteria: (i) arrival by ambulance; (ii) vomiting; (iii) a diastolic blood pressure of 100 mmHg or above; and (iv) age 45 years or above. The rule was found to be 100% sensitive (95% CI: 97–100) and 36% specific (95% CI: 34–39) for the detection of SAH. This data was published in abstract form only, and as of the writing of this book no validation has been reported. In addition, the use of 'arrival by ambulance' as a criterion in any decision rule considerably limits the validity and generalizability of the rule.

SAH is infrequently found on LP after a negative head CT. However, when patients are at high risk for SAH, a LP is certainly indicated. Given that a head CT does not completely rule out SAH, physicians often have to make the difficult decision of whether to perform a LP when SAH is considered but the head CT is negative. Elements that often influence this decision include the pre-test probability, the complication rate of LP, patient desire, and the concern over missing a potentially life-threatening disease. While LP has been shown to be a safe procedure, it still carries a relatively high rate of postdural headaches (up to 20–40% of cases). Up to 35% of patients will also experience low back pain. Also, in a busy ED, performing an LP can take considerable time by the emergency physician and can thus increase the length of stay in the ED.

Clinical question

"What is the sensitivity of noncontrast head CT for subarachnoid hemorrhage?"
The operating characteristic of sensitivity for noncontrast head CT for SAH has been described in many studies. The major difference between these studies involves the type of CT scanner used. While earlier papers employed single-row CT scans to investigate nontraumatic SAH, more recent studies have reported data on multidetector-row CT scans and have reported higher sensitivity.

One of the first studies reporting data on nontraumatic SAH investigated the need for LP in patients that presented within the first 12 h of headache onset and that had normal neurological examinations.[2] They enrolled a consecutive series of 175 patients where SAH was clinically suspected. All patients had a noncontrast head CT followed by a LP (at 12 h or more after the headache onset) if the head CT was negative. The CT was positive for SAH in 117 patients (67%); of the 58 patients with negative head CTs, CSF analysis revealed SAH in two patients (3%; 95% CI: 0.4–12). In both of those cases, there was evidence of a ruptured aneurysm. Therefore, in two out of 119 patients with SAH, the head CT was negative for a test sensitivity of 98% (95% CI: 92–100).

Another group studied data from patients with SAH from 1988 to 1994.[3] They excluded patients who were age less than two years old and those that had a history of head trauma within 24 h of onset of symptoms. They stratified patients into two groups based on symptom duration (<24 h and >24 h). They used a third-generation CT scanner for all scans in the study and all patients with negative head CTs received a diagnostic LP. In 181 patients, they determined the sensitivity of CT to be 93% for patients whose head CT was performed with 24 h of symptom onset, and 84% for patients whose head CT was performed after 24 h for an overall sensitivity of 92%. This indicates that there is a spectrum bias that occurs with the use of CT scanning in SAH where as time goes by the sensitivity decreases.

Another study investigated the use of third-generation CT scanners in patients with SAH over a three year period.[4] Similar to the previous study, patients received a noncontrast head CT followed by a LP if the CT was negative, and patients were stratified according to time of onset (<12 h and >12 h). Of 140 patients with SAH, the authors reported 100% sensitivity (95% CI: 95–100) in the 80 patients that were tested within 12 h of symptom onset and 82% (95% CI: 70–90) in patients tested after 12 h of symptom onset. They found that 11 out of 140 (8%) patients had a positive CSF for SAH after a negative head CT.

One of the only prospective studies examining this issue studied patients who presented with the 'worst headache of my life' and who received LP if their CT was negative.[5] Of the 107 patients enrolled, SAH was detected by CT in 18 patients (17%). Two patients (3%; 95% CI: 0–9) had SAH detected by LP after a negative head CT.

The most recent study investigating this issue used a fifth-generation multidetector-row CT scanner.[6] Of 177 ED patients studied over a one-year period that had a CT followed by a LP, they found that none had a negative head CT and a positive LP.

Comment

Among the studies presented here there are some major limitations that need to be pointed out. Most of the studies are retrospective and did not follow patients who were discharged home without any testing or with just a negative head CT. This is important because there may have been cases of SAH that were missed either because no testing was performed or because no LP was performed. Performances of the diagnostic tests would be expected to be different to those reported had potentially missed cases been considered.

There were also considerable differences in the prevalence of disease among the populations studied, the highest being 67%. Certainly, in our practice such a high prevalence does not adequately characterize the patients that are assessed for SAH. This selection bias may affect the test sensitivity in a number of ways. It may underestimate it considerably because patients who had a negative head CT only and did not receive the gold standard test, either because the physician or the patient did not feel that the test was indicated, may dramatically increase the denominator for whom SAH was considered in the differential diagnosis. It is also possible that it could go the other way, where some patients with SAH were sent home without any testing. Most of the studies did not follow patients and did not enroll a broad cohort of patients with headache to exclude either of these possibilities.

However, what is clear from these studies is the evidence of a spectrum bias, where test sensitivity decreases as time passes from the onset of acute headache. There were also variable definitions for a positive LP. Because there are no widely accepted, validated criteria for a positive LP it can be difficult to distinguish a traumatic tap—whereby red blood cells from the mechanical process of performing the procedure get into the CSF—from a truly positive tap. Finally, fifth-generation multidetector-row CT scanners seem be more accurate than earlier third-generation scanners in picking up SAH, indicating that test sensitivity may be higher in centers using the former. In addition, many of these studies had small sample sizes and were performed at only one center, both of which limits the generalizability of some these findings.

In largest study on missed SAH, the most common reason for missed diagnosis was the failure to order a head CT.[7] In patients that present with the 'worst headache of their life', or when a patient who does not usually get headaches presents with a new severe headache, or a patient with chronic headaches presents with a change in their headache symptoms, then noncontrast head CT is a reasonable diagnostic test if it is available. In our practice, the choice to perform LP on patients is highly dependent on the pre-test probability for disease. Given the high risk of complications, including postdural headache and lower back pain, in centers where multidetector-row CT is available, it may be reasonable practice to defer LP in cases where there is a low pre-test probability.

References

1. Perry, J.J., Stiell, I.G., Wells, G.A., *et al.* (2006) A clinical decision rule to safely rule out subarachnoid hemorrhage in acute headache patients in the emergency department. *Academic Emergency Medicine* **13**: S9.
2. van der Wee, N., Rinkel, G.J. and Hasan, D. (1995) Detection of subarachnoid haemorrhage on early CT: is lumbar puncture still needed after a negative scan? *Journal of Neurology, Neurosurgery and Psychiatry* **58**: 357–359.
3. Sames, T.A., Storrow, A.B., Finkelstein, J.A. and Magoon, M.R. (1996) Sensitivity of new-generation computed tomography in subarachnoid hemorrhage. *Academic Emergency Medicine* **3**: 16–20.
4. Sidman, R., Connolly, E. and Lemke, T. (1996) Subarachnoid hemorrhage diagnosis: lumbar puncture is still needed when the computed tomography scan is normal. *Academic Emergency Medicine* **3**: 827–831.
5. Morgenstern, L.B., Luna-Gonzales, H. and Huber, J.C., Jr, *et al.* (1998) Worst headache and subarachnoid hemorrhage: prospective, modern computed tomography and spinal fluid analysis. *Annals of Emergency Medicine* **32**: 297–304.
6. Boesiger, B.M. and Shiber, J.R. (2005) Subarachnoid hemorrhage diagnosis by computed tomography and lumbar puncture: are fifth generation CT scanners better at identifying subarachnoid hemorrhage? *Journal of Emergency Medicine* **29**: 23–27.
7. Kowalski, R.G., Classen, J. and Kreiter, K.T. (2004) Initial misdiagnosis and outcome after subarachnoid hemorrhage. *Journal of the American Medical Association* **291**: 866–869.

Chapter 36 **Acute Stroke**

Highlights

- Rapid evaluation of patients with acute stroke using noncontrast head computed tomography (CT) scanning is critical in differentiating hemorrhagic versus ischemic stroke and in identifying patients that may be candidates for intravenous thrombolysis (within three hours of symptom onset).
- Magnetic resonance imaging (MRI) with diffusion-weighted imaging (DWI) is more sensitive (~97%) than noncontrast head CT for detecting ischemic strokes.
- Noncontrast head CT and MRI can both accurately differentiate ischemic from hemorrhagic stroke, but MRI can provide more information on microhemorrhages.
- Noncontrast CT remains the standard brain imaging study for the initial emergency department (ED) evaluation of patients with acute stroke symptoms; however, MRI may gain favor as it becomes more widely available.

Background

Stroke is the third leading cause of death in the US and the leading cause of disability. Rapid bedside and radiological evaluation in cases of acute stroke within 6 h of symptom onset are critical in the assessment of patients that are potentially eligible for intravenous and intra-arterial thrombolysis with tissue plasminogen activator (tPA). In acute ischemic stroke, the central event is an acute vascular occlusion (Fig. 36.1); however, 15% of strokes are hemorrhagic (Fig. 36.2). Hemorrhagic strokes treated with tPA do not benefit from

Evidence-Based Emergency Care: Diagnostic Testing and Clinical Decision Rules. By J.M. Pines and W.W. Everett. Published 2008 by Blackwell Publishing, ISBN: 978-14051-5400-0.

thrombolysis; indeed this can worsen bleeding and can be lethal. Today, intravenous thrombolysis is the treatment of choice in patients that have ischemic lesions involving greater than one third of the middle cerebral artery territory, no incidence of intracranial hemorrhage presenting within 3 h of the onset of symptoms, and no other contraindications for tPA usage. Traditionally, noncontrast head CT is the first imaging modality in acute stroke in the ED. By using noncontrast head CT we are able to differentiate between hemorrhagic and ischemic stroke, and can also exclude other potential causes of acute neurological symptoms. Multimodal MRI with DWI is one of the more advanced imaging techniques that are frequently performed after CT scanning because it is considered to be a more accurate diagnostic test for stroke. The primary clinical concerns regarding the use of MRI with DWI as a solitary test are: (i) its reduced ability to detect intracranial hemorrhage in the setting of acute stroke; (ii) the poorer clinical access for potentially unstable patients; (iii) longer testing times; and (iv) the poor availability of rapid MRI.

Clinical question

"What is the sensitivity of diagnostic modalities (head CT and MRI) in acute stroke, and does MRI miss acute intracranial hemorrhages?"
A recent review of articles has been published in which noncontrast head CT was compared to MRI with DWI in acute stroke patients in order to calculate sensitivity and specificity values.[1] The authors included articles where both

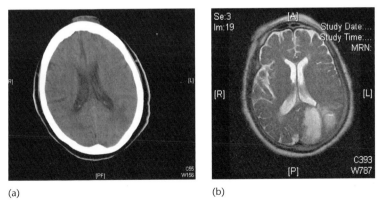

(a) (b)

Figure 36.1 Noncontrast head computed tomography showing ischemic stroke in the left posterior cerebral artery region (a), which was confirmed by magnetic resonance imaging (b).

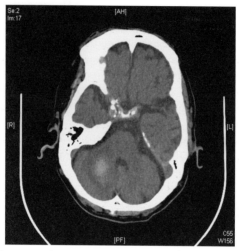

Figure 36.2 Noncontrast head computed tomography showing a right cerebellar hemorrhage.

head CT and MRI were performed within 6–7 h of the onset of clinical symptoms. A total of eight studies met the authors' inclusion criteria.

The largest study to be reviewed by these authors was a retrospective chart review of 733 patients seen in the ED for signs and symptoms of acute stroke.[2] The inclusion criterion was that imaging was performed within 6 h of arrival in the ED. Patients were excluded if they were diagnosed with a transient ischemic attack (i.e. resolving symptoms). Of 691 patients, 509 had a noncontrast head CT and 122 had MRI with DWI. The gold standard for diagnosis was a primary discharge diagnosis of stroke. The study reported a sensitivity for noncontrast head CT of 40%, and a sensitivity for MRI with DWI of 97%. Specificity was 92% for both modalities. The positive predictive value (PPV) was 96% for both head CT and MRI with DWI. The negative predictive value (NPV) was 23% for head CT and 77% for MRI with DWI. This study was limited by its retrospective nature, the presence of incomplete records, and the potential bias in the selection of which patients received both studies.

The authors went on to review seven other smaller studies (ranging in sample size from 17 to 54), most with considerable methodological issues including delays between head CT and MRI with DWI, and variability in the inclusion criteria, gold standards used, and in the blinding of reviewers.[3–9] They then combined data from all eight studies (despite the variable inclusion criteria) to calculate sensitivity, specificity, PPV, and NPV values for each modality. For MRI with DWI, the sensitivity was 97% (95% CI: 94–98), specificity 100% (95% CI: 88–100), PPV 100% (95% CI: 98–100), and NPV 91% (95% CI: 75–98). The sensitivity of head CT was 47% (95% CI: 43–51), specificity 93% (95% CI: 85–97), PPV 97% (95% CI: 94–99), and NPV 23% (95% CI: 19–28).

Another more recent prospective study compared MRI with DWI to non-contrast CT in the ED in a single center in patients with suspected stroke.[10] The scans were interpreted independently by four separate radiologists who were blinded to clinical information. In 356 patients, 217 had a final diagnosis of acute stroke. MRI detected acute stroke (both ischemic and hemorrhagic) and chronic hemorrhage more frequently than CT ($P < 0.0001$, for all comparisons). However, in the detection of acute intracranial hemorrhage, MRI was similar to CT. MRI and CT detected acute ischemic stroke in 164 out of 356 patients (46%; 95% CI: 41–51) and 35 out of 356 patients (10%; 95% CI: 7–14), respectively. A subset analysis was performed on patients who were scanned within 3 h of the onset of symptoms. In those patients, MRI and CT detected acute ischemic stroke in 41 out of 90 patients (46%; 95% CI: 35–56) and 6 out of 90 patients (7%; 95% CI: 3–14), respectively. Using the final clinical diagnosis as the gold standard, they reported a sensitivity of 83% (95% CI: 78–88) for MRI and 26% (95% CI: 20–32) for CT. The authors concluded that MRI was better than CT in terms of its ability to detect acute ischemia. There were no differences in detecting acute and chronic hemorrhage. They concluded that MRI should be the preferred test for patients with suspected stroke.

Other studies have confirmed that MRI with DWI is as sensitive as CT scanning for detecting acute intracranial hemorrhage. Fiebach *et al.* performed a multicenter study to test how accurate MRI was in the detection of acute intracranial hemorrhage in patients with suspected stroke.[11] They compared MRI images from 62 patients with intracranial hemorrhages and 62 without intracranial hemorrhages, all of whom were imaged within 6 h of symptom onset, using CT as the gold standard. Experienced readers of MRI were able to detect intracranial hemorrhage in all cases (100% sensitivity; 95% CI: 97–100).

Kidwell *et al.* also compared the accuracy of MRI to that of CT in detecting intracranial hemorrhage in patients within 6 h of onset of the acute focal symptoms of stroke in two centers.[12] Patients presenting underwent MRI followed by a noncontrast CT and scans were read by four blinded readers. The authors stopped the study early after only 200 patients were enrolled as a result of an interim analysis where they found that MRI was detecting cases of hemorrhagic transformation that were not detected on CT scans. MRI was positive in 71 patients with any hemorrhage and CT was positive in 29

($P < 0.001$). There was no difference in the ability of MRI and CT to diagnose acute hemorrhage. Acute hemorrhage was detected in 25 patients on both MRI and CT; however, in four different patients acute hemorrhage was detected on MRI but not CT. In three of the patients, regions that were interpreted as an acute hemorrhage on CT scans were read as chronic hemorrhage on MRI. There was one patient in whom subarachnoid hemorrhage was seen on CT scans but not on MRI. Chronic hemorrhage (microbleeds) that was not seen on CT scan was visualized by MRI in 49 patients. The authors concluded that MRI was as accurate as CT scanning in detecting acute hemorrhage in patients with acute focal symptoms of stroke, and was more accurate than CT in detecting chronic intracranial hemorrhage.

Comment

In emergency care, the current standard in cases of acute stroke is non-contrast head CT to determine the presence of intracranial hemorrhage, detect large strokes, and potentially exclude other neurological causes for stroke symptoms. Head CT and clinical evaluation are the standards by which the decision to use thrombolysis is typically made. Because head CT has limited sensitivity, thrombolysis is used in up to one fifth of the cases of stroke mimics. In most instances then this is followed by MRI with DWI, which is a more sensitive test for acute stroke. However, this modality has limited availability, higher cost, takes longer to perform, and requires a higher degree of patient participation. MRI with DWI is also more sensitive than head CT in identifying large-volume strokes, which are at increased risk of hemorrhagic transformation and are also more sensitive at detecting chronic intracranial hemorrhage.

A primary historical concern with the use of only MRI with DWI in acute stroke was that head CT was more sensitive at detecting acute intracranial hemorrhage. However, recent studies with newer MRI technology have virtually disproved this. In the future, improvements in the availability of MRI may make it the only test needed for stroke assessment in the ED.

References

1. Davis, D.P., Robertson, T. and Imbesi, S.G. (2006) Diffusion-weighted magnetic resonance imaging versus computed tomography in the diagnosis of acute ischemic stroke. *Journal of Emergency Medicine* **31**: 269–277.
2. Mullins, M.E., Schaefer, P.W., Sorensen, A.G., *et al.* (2002) CT and conventional and diffusion-weighted MR imaging in acute stroke: study in 691 patients at presentation to the emergency department. *Radiology* **224**: 353–359.

3. Fiebach, J., Jansen, O., Schellinger, P., *et al.* (2001) Comparison of CT with diffusion-weighted MRI in patients with hyperacute stroke. *Neuroradiology* **43**: 628–632.

4. Fiebach, J.B., Schellinger, P.D., Jansen, O., *et al.* (2002) CT and diffusion-weighted MR imaging in randomized order. *Stroke* **33**: 2206–2210.

5. Urbach, H., Flacke, S., Keller, E., *et al.* (2000) Detectability and detection rate of acute cerebral hemisphere infarcts on CT and diffusion-weighted MRI. *Neuroradiology* **42**: 722–727.

6. Lansberg, M.G., Albers, G.W., Beaulieu, C. and Marks, M.P. (2000) Comparison of diffusion-weighted MRI and CT in acute stroke. *Neurology* **54**: 1557–1561.

7. Gonzales, R.G., Schaefer, P.W., Buonanno, F.S., *et al.* (1999) Diffusion-weighted MR imaging: diagnostic accuracy in patients imaged within 6 hours of stroke symptom onset. *Radiology* **210**: 155–162.

8. Barber, P.A., Darby, D.G., Desmond, P.M., *et al.* (1999) Identification of major ischemic change, diffusion-weighted imaging versus computed tomography. *Stroke* **30**: 2059–2065.

9. Saur, D., Kucinski, T., Grzyska, U., *et al.* (2003) Sensitivity and interrater agreement of CT and diffusion-weighted MR imaging in hyperacute stroke. AJNR *American Journal of Neuroradiology* **24**: 878–885.

10. Chalela, J.A., Kidwell, C.S., Nentwich, L.M., *et al.* (2007) Magnetic resonance imaging and computed tomography in emergency assessment of patients with suspected acute stroke: a prospective comparison. *Lancet* **369**: 293–298.

11. Fiebach, J.B., Schellinger, P.D., Gass, A., *et al.* (2004) Stroke magnetic resonance imaging is accurate in hyperacute intracerebral hemorrhage: a multicenter study on the validity of stroke imaging. *Stroke* **35**: 502–506.

12. Kidwell, C.S., Chalela, J.A., Saver, J.L., *et al.* (2004) Comparison of MRI and CT for detection of acute intracerebral hemorrhage. *Journal of the American Medical Association* **292**(15): 1823–1830.

Miscellaneous: Ophthalmology, Hematology, Rheumatology, and Pulmonology

Chapter 37 **Pulmonary Embolism and Deep Vein Thrombosis**

Highlights

- Deep venous thrombosis (DVT) and pulmonary embolism (PE) are potentially lethal conditions that can present atypically.
- Scoring systems like the Wells criteria, the Geneva score, and the Pulmonary Embolism Research Consortium (PERC) rule can offer a guide for clinicians as to the likelihood of thromboembolic disease.
- Diagnostic evaluation involves risk assessment coupled with D-dimer testing for low to very low-risk patients.
- Imaging studies include venous compression ultrasound for DVT and chest computed tomography angiography (CTA) plus venous-phase multidetector computed tomography venography (CTV) for pulmonary embolism.

Background

Diagnosing DVT and PE, also known together as venous thromboembolic (VTE) disease, represents a challenge in emergency care because both can present with nonspecific symptoms and both can be potentially lethal. Accurate and timely identification of patients with DVT and PE in the emergency department (ED) can minimize complications and morbidity. However, both DVT and PE are relatively rare entities—ones that are often sought but infrequently found. Approximately 84 in 100 000 patients per year develop DVT and between 100 and 200 in 100 000 patients per year develop PE. The challenge in diagnosing DVT and PE in the ED is the appropriate selection of patients for diagnostic testing and risk stratification based on clinical findings. While many tests are available for DVT and PE for ED patients, there is a large literature on this topic—mostly directed at the determination

Evidence-Based Emergency Care: Diagnostic Testing and Clinical Decision Rules. By J.M. Pines and W.W. Everett. Published 2008 by Blackwell Publishing, ISBN: 978-14051-5400-0.

of pre-test probabilities using clinical decision rules, and the calculation of sensitivity and specificity for a diagnostic test. The following is not meant to be a comprehensive review of all aspects of the diagnosis of DVT and PE in the ED; rather, it is a compilation of clinically relevant questions and studies providing objective data for specific research questions.

There are multiple tests for PE, including the D-dimer test (performed as an enzyme-linked immunosorbant assay (ELISA) or whole-blood assay), chest computed tomography (CT), ventilation/perfusion (V/Q) scan, and pulmonary angiogram. The choice of test is traditionally made following assessment of the pre-test probability of disease based on objective clinical criteria, where lower risk patients can receive D-dimers to rule out PE and higher risk patients traditionally receive more tests, which have higher sensitivities, such as a chest CT or V/Q scan. Because the pulmonary angiogram, long considered the gold standard test for PE, has a 1.5% incidence of serious complications as a result of the test itself, it is rarely used to make a diagnosis and/or guide patient management unless absolutely necessary.

Venous non-compressibility assessed using ultrasound is the major diagnostic criterion for venous thrombosis (Fig. 37.1). However, compression ultrasound is not specific or sensitive enough for detecting DVT in patients with asymptomatic proximal DVT or in patients with DVT in the calf. It also has limited accuracy in cases of chronic DVT. The use of ultrasound is further limited in patients who are obese or who have edema. In general, despite its limitations, leg compression ultrasound is used to detect DVT in the ED. Traditionally, only the proximal veins (from the femoral veins down to the calf where they join the popliteal veins) are studied. DVTs usually start in the calf and, in symptomatic DVT, more than 80% of the time this involves the popliteal vein and more proximal leg veins. In patients with calf DVTs that may not be detected on the first ED ultrasound, about 20% will extend more proximally within about a week. Non-extending calf DVTs very rarely cause PE while proximal DVTs are at much higher risk for propagation and hence for causing PE.

Clinical question one

"How sensitive is ultrasound in detecting DVT?"
A recent review of non-invasive methods for the diagnosis of first and recurrent DVT was performed to study the diagnostic sensitivity of ultrasound.[1] The authors used contrast venography as the gold standard for the detection of DVT and included only prospective cohort studies and randomized clinical trials. Combined data from individual studies were assessed using a random-effects model. In this pooled analysis the sensitivity of venous

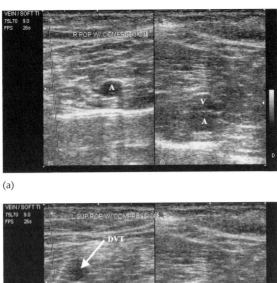

(a)

(b)

Figure 37.1 Compression ultrasound of the right and left popliteal vessels. The screen is split to show the noncompressed normal anatomy on the right-hand side and the compressed anatomy on the left-hand side. The left popliteal vein is noncompressible and represents a venous thrombus. A, artery; V, vein. (Courtesy of Anthony Dean, MD).

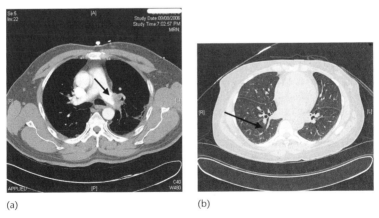

(a)   (b)

Figure 37.2 (a and b) Chest computed tomography images showing an acute pulmonary embolus (arrow).

ultrasound for symptomatic proximal DVT was 97% (95% CI: 96–98%) and for symptomatic distal DVT it was 73% (95% CI: 54–93%). The authors concluded that venous ultrasound is the most accurate non-invasive test for symptomatic DVT.

Clinical question two

"What are the sensitivity and specificity of D-dimer tests in the diagnosis of DVT?" Using a negative D-dimer test to exclude DVT is highly dependent on the type of assay employed, which can be of either high or moderate sensitivity. As the sensitivity of the assay drops, so too does the ability to use a negative test to rule out DVT. While there are many commercially available D-dimer assays, there are two specific methods that have been studied extensively: the ELISA and the whole-blood assay. Among the different assays, there is wide variation in the sensitivity, normal reference ranges, and cut off points. A recently published meta-analysis of different D-dimer assays reported a sensitivity of 95% or above for ELISAs and certain immunoturbidimetric tests, but also reported a low specificity (≥40%) at a cut off of 500 ng/dL or above.[2] Other D-dimer assays such as whole blood and quantitative latex agglutination assays are less sensitive, with a reported rate of about 85%, but are more specific (approximately 65%).

A recent systematic review examined this question by looking at 14 studies that included a total of 8000 patients.[3] Using the Wells criteria the prevalence of DVT was 5.0, 17, and 53% in the low, medium, and high-risk groups, respectively (Table 37.1). Pooled analysis revealed that the sensitivity and specificity of the D-dimer test were 88% (95% CI: 81–92) and 72% (95% CI: 65–78) for the low probability group, 90% (95% CI: 80–95) and 58% (95% CI: 49–67) for the medium probability group, and 92% (95% CI: 85–96) and 45% (95% CI: 37–52) for the high probability group. This does indicate some spectrum bias in D-dimer testing in DVT. However, before using D-dimer testing to rule out DVT, care should be taken to understand the test characteristics of the specific assay used by the laboratory in your hospital.

Clinical question three

"What are the Wells criteria for assessing the pre-test probability of DVT and PE?" The initial derivation of the Wells criteria for PE involved the development of a simplified scoring system to calculate a pre-test probability in patients with suspected PE.[4] The authors used a randomly selected sample of 80% of patients with suspected PE that had participated in a prospective cohort

Table 37.1 Pooled analysis of the performance characteristics of the D-dimer test for ruling out deep vein thrombosis from Wells et al.[3]

Specific measure	Pre-test probability		
	Low	Moderate	High
Sensitivity, %	88 (81–92)	90 (80–95)	92 (85–96)
Specificity, %	72 (65–78)	58 (49–67)	45 (37–52)
NPV	99 (98–99)	96 (94–97)	84 (77–89)
PPV	17 (13–20)	32 (25–41)	66 (56–75)

NPV, negative predictive value; PPV, positive predictive value.

study of patients and had received D-dimer testing (SimpleRED test), and performed logistic regression analysis using 40 clinical variables to create a clinical prediction rule. They created cut off points for the new rule and devised two separate scoring systems. The first classified patients as having low, moderate, or high probability of PE, and the second created two categories, PE likely and PE unlikely. The goal in the second system was that patients who were PE unlikely and had a negative D-dimer test would have a PE prevalence of less than 2%. The authors then applied these probabilities to the remaining 20% of the sample (to validate the scoring system). Seven variables ended up being predictive of PE and were termed the Wells criteria for PE (see Table 37.2).

The interpreted point totals did not include D-dimer testing. 'PE unlikely' was assigned to patients with a score of four points or less. Without the use

Table 37.2 The Wells criteria for assessing the pre-test probability of suspected pulmonary embolism (PE) from Wells et al.[4]

Clinical factor	Point score*
Clinical DVT (objective leg swelling, tenderness)	3.0
Heart rate ≥100 bpm	1.5
Immobilization >3 days or surgery in previous 4 weeks	1.5
Previous DVT/PE	1.5
Hemoptysis	1.0
Malignancy	1.0
PE as likely or more likely than alternative diagnosis	3.0

DVT, deep venous thrombosis.
* Interpretation of point score: <2 points, low risk (mean probability: 3.6%); 2–6 points, moderate risk (mean probability: 20.5%); ≥6 points, high risk (mean probability: 66.7%).

of D-dimer testing, the prevalence of PE in those whose score was greater than four was 7.8%. However, when the D-dimer was negative, the rate of PE was only 2.2% (95% CI: 1.0–4.0) in the derivation dataset and 1.7% in the validation dataset. Using a cut-off of two points or less, a negative D-dimer test resulted in a PE rate of 1.5% (95% CI: 0.4–3.7) in the derivation dataset and 2.7% (95% CI: 0.3–9.0) in the validation dataset, and only occurred in 29% of patients. The authors concluded that a combination of a score of four or less and a negative D-dimer test may have a negative predictive value where safe discharge is possible in patients with suspected PE.

Dr. Wells and colleagues also derived and validated a similar rule for DVT (see Table 37.3).[5] In the validation study, all patients had ultrasonography and venography. In 529 patients, the Wells criteria predicted the prevalence of DVT in high (85%), medium (33%) and low-risk (5%) cases.

Clinical question four

"What is the Geneva score for PE and how does this compare to the Wells score?"
The Geneva score is a system that clinicians can use to risk-stratify patients with potential PE, similar to the Wells score. The original scoring system was limited in that it required arterial blood gas analysis, which is painful and unnecessary in low-risk patients. The revised Geneva score was recently published and this does not include arterial blood gas analysis.[6] This scoring system also does not require an assessment by the physician regarding whether PE is the leading diagnosis, as in the Wells score.

The revised Geneva score was derived in 965 consecutive patients that were evaluated for PE according to a standardized protocol. A total of 23% of

Table 37.3 The Wells criteria for deep vein thrombosis (DVT) from Wells *et al.*[5]

Clinical feature	Score*
Active cancer (current treatment or within 6 months or palliative)	1
Paralysis, paresis, or recent immobilization	1
Recently bedridden for >3 days or major surgery within 4 weeks	1
Localised calf tenderness	1
Entire leg swollen	1
Calf swelling >3 cm compared with the asymptomatic leg (10 cm below tibial tuberosity)	1
Pitting edema in the symptomatic leg	1
Collateral superficial veins (non-varicose)	1
Alternative diagnosis as likely or greater than that of DVT	–2

* Interpretation of score: high risk, ≥3 points; moderate risk, 1–2 points; low risk, ≤0 points.

patients in the derivation cohort and 26% in the validation cohort had PE. The area under the receiver operating characteristic (ROC) was 0.74 (95% CI: 0.70–0.78) in both the derivation and validation datasets. The revised Geneva score also performed well in an external validation cohort of 756 patients (see Tables 37.4 and 37.5).

Clinical question five

"Which patients require testing for PE and can the Pulmonary Embolism Research Consortium (PERC) rule aid in making this decision?"
Overuse of the D-dimer test to screen for possible PE can have negative consequences due to its low specificity. Because patients with elevated D-dimers get CT scans to rule out PE and the number of negative CTs for PE is high, having the ability to select which patients need testing to rule out PE would be clinically helpful. A study by Kline *et al.* aimed to derive and test clinical criteria to justify not ordering a D-dimer test on ED patients.[7] They

Table 37.4 The revised Geneva score from Pierre *et al.*[6]

	Points
Risk factors:	
Age >65 years	1
Previous DVT or PE	3
Surgery or fracture within one month	2
Active malignancy	2
Symptoms:	
Unilateral lower limb pain	3
Hemoptysis	2
Clinical signs:	
Heart rate 75–94 bpm	3
Heart rate ≥95 bpm	5
Pain on lower limb deep vein palpation and unilateral edema	4

DVT, deep venous thrombosis; PE, pulmonary embolism.

Table 37.5 The revised Geneva score: classification according to points

Total points	Risk	Prevalence of PE*
0–3	Low	7.9%
4–10	Intermediate	28%
≥11	High	74%

* In the validation cohort.

constructed a prediction rule, called the PERC rule, in 3148 ED patients in order to identify those at such low risk that they would not require any testing at all for PE. The authors sought to find variables that were associated with the absence of PE. In the derivation study, the prevalence of PE was 11%. The final model derived consisted of eight criteria. If all of the following are negative, the patient does not require testing for PE and PE can be ruled out on clinical grounds:

- age less than 50 years;
- pulse less than 100 bpm;
- oxygen saturation greater than 94%;
- absence of unilateral leg swelling;
- no hemoptysis;
- no recent trauma or surgery;
- no history of DVT or PE; and
- no hormone use.

A validation set included 1427 low-risk patients, 8% of which had PE. The rule was negative (i.e. did not meet any of the criteria) in 25% of them. Among those who were PERC rule-negative, the proportion with PE was only 1.4% (95% CI: 0.4–3.2). The authors concluded that these low-risk patients did not need a test for PE. When the same rule was applied retrospectively to a cohort with a 25% prevalence of PE, 6.7% had PE.[8] At the 2007 Society for Academic Emergency Medicine meeting, Dr. Kline presented a multicenter validation of the PERC rule and validated the results across multiple settings. The formal peer-reviewed publication of this work is still pending at the time of writing this book.

Clinical question six

"Can CT of the chest be used as a diagnostic endpoint in patients at high risk of PE?"

First generation CT scanners demonstrated poor sensitivity (70%) for detecting PE. However, in the past few years multidetector-row CT scanning has been piloted as a potential replacement to pulmonary angiography (Fig. 37.2). In a prospective study of 756 patients that were referred to the ED with a suspicion of PE (prevalence of 26%), 524 patients that had either a high clinical probability, or a low or medium clinical probability and a positive D-dimer test (ELISA), received both a lower extremity ultrasound and a multidetector-row chest CT.[9] A total of three out of 324 patients had a proximal DVT on ultrasound and a negative chest CT (0.9%). At the three-month follow-up, the overall risk of DVT and PE was estimated to be 1.5% (95% CI: 0.8–3.0) if the D-dimer assay and CT scanning were the only tests used to rule out PE. This study suggests that multidetector-row CT scanning and the D-dimer test can be used alone, without employing pulmonary angiogram, in low or medium-risk patients. These data have been corroborated by another study of 3306 patients that included mostly outpatients with suspected PE.[10] Patients that were high risk according to the Wells score had a chest CT, and those who were considered to be low or medium risk were assessed by D-dimer testing. Patients with elevated D-dimer levels underwent a chest CT. The three-month DVT and PE risk in patients that were not treated on the basis of a negative chest CT was 1.1% (95% CI: 0.6–1.9). This was independent of the pre-test probability for PE.

Comment

Over the past ten years the assessment of ED patients for possible DVT and PE has changed considerably. There is a significant amount of information available regarding the characteristics of laboratory tests and imaging studies, making the application of evidence-based medicine at the bedside a practicable reality. Venous compression ultrasound has replaced contrast venography in the evaluation of DVT. The D-dimer assay is also useful in evaluating patients that are at low risk of DVT; however, there is spectrum bias and the test sensitivity only reaches 88% in the lowest risk group. There is good evidence that the D-dimer assay can be used safely in patients who are at low or medium risk of PE, and that multidetector-row chest CT is a safe way to evaluate higher risk presentations.

The recently published results of the PIOPED II study, which was a multicenter trial of CTA combined with venous-phase multidetector CTV, reported that in 824 patients CTA was 83% sensitive and 96% specific for the diagnosis of PE.[11] In about 10% of patients the results of CTA-CTV were inconclusive because of poor image quality, but it was shown that CTA-CTV was 90% sensitive and 95% specific for PE. The authors concluded that in patients with suspected PE, the use of multidetector-row CTA with CTV has a higher sensitivity than CTA alone. However, they did warn that additional testing should be performed when the clinical probability is not consistent with imaging results. These results indicate to us that for higher risk cases, multidetector-row CTA with CTV should be the test of choice, if it is available. However, when patients are at very high risk of PE, based on a clinical scoring system like the Wells score, a negative CTA-CTV should not be used as the diagnostic endpoint, rather the gold standard pulmonary angiogram should be performed.

The question of how to select patients that do not require testing for PE is challenging, because in order to achieve a high negative predictive value this needs to be applied to a very low-risk population. Deciding whether or not to consider a patient at any risk for PE occurs much more frequently than discriminating between medium and high-risk patients. The PERC rule seems to perform well in the initial derivation and unpublished validation study. In the future, as further studies on the PERC rule are published in ED patients at low risk for PE (<15% prevalence), then this scoring system may become a useful addition to everyday practice. Applying this rule to a higher risk group, however, should be performed with caution because the number of false negatives may be too high for practical use.

Finally, in all these studies, when the gold standard test (pulmonary angiogram) is not undertaken or when the D-dimer test is used for low and medium-risk patients, there is always a chance that a patient will be sent home with DVT or PE. Where we draw the line—that is, where we set our standard for risk tolerance with our patients—is very physician-specific and practice-specific. You should ensure that the risks and benefits of the various diagnostic strategies are explained thoroughly to your patients and they should be involved in the decision-making process for this highly challenging disease.

References

1. Kearon, C., Julian, J.A., Newman, T.E., *et al.* (1998) Noninvasive diagnosis of deep vein thrombosis. *Annals of Internal Medicine* **128**: 663–677.
2. Stein, P.D., Hull, R.D., Patel, K.C., *et al.* (2004) D-dimer for the exclusion of acute venous thrombosis and pulmonary embolism. A systematic review. *Annals of Internal Medicine* **140**: 589–602.
3. Wells, P.S., Owen, C., Doucette, S., *et al.* (2006) Does this patient have deep vein thrombosis? *Journal of the American Medical Association* **295**: 199–207.
4. Wells, P.S., Anderson, D.R., Rodger, M., *et al.* (2000) Derivation of a simple clinical model to categorize patients' probability of pulmonary embolism: increasing the model's utility with the SimpliRED D-dimer. *Thrombosis and Haemostasis* **83**: 416–420.
5. Wells, P.S., Hirsh, J., Anderson, D.R., *et al.* (1995) Accuracy of clinical assessment of deep-vein thrombosis. *Lancet* **345**(8961): 1326–1330.
6. Perrier, A., Roy, P.M., Aujesky, D., *et al.* (2004) Diagnosing pulmonary embolism in outpatients with clinical assessment, D-dimer measurement, venous ultrasound, and helical computed tomography: a multicenter management study. *American Journal of Medicine* **116**: 291–299.
7. Kline, J.A., Mitchell, A.M., Kabrhel, C., *et al.* (2004) Clinical criteria to prevent unnecessary diagnostic testing in emergency department patients with suspected pulmonary embolism. *Journal of Thrombosis and Haemostasis* **2**: 1247–1255.
8. Righini, M., Le Gal, G., Perrier, A. and Bounameaux, H. (2005) More on: clinical criteria to prevent unnecessary diagnostic testing in emergency department

patients with suspected pulmonary embolism. *Journal of Thrombosis and Haemostasis* **3**:188–189.

 9. Perrier, A., Roy, P.M., Sanchez, O., *et al.* (2005) Multidetector-row computed tomography in suspected pulmonary embolism. *New England Journal of Medicine* **352**: 1760–1768.

10. van Belle, A., Buller, H.R., Huisman, M.V., *et al.* (2006) Effectiveness of managing suspected pulmonary embolism using an algorithm combining clinical probability, D-dimer testing, and computed tomography. *Journal of the American Medical Association* **295**: 172–179.

11. Stein, P.D., Fowler, S.E., Goodman, L.R., *et al.* (2006) Multidetector computed tomography for acute pulmonary embolism. *New England Journal of Medicine* **354**: 2317–2322.

Chapter 38 **Temporal Arteritis**

> **Highlights**
>
> - Temporal arteritis typically presents as an acute unilateral headache in older adults and can cause permanent visual impairment.
> - Definitive diagnosis is achieved with temporal artery biopsy.
> - An abnormal erythrocyte sedimentation rate (ESR) is highly sensitive and serves as a good screening tool for this disease.

Background

Temporal arteritis is an inflammatory condition characterized by focal, granulomatous changes to branches of the carotid artery that leads to vessel damage, stenosis, and occlusion. Histopathologic findings from temporal artery biopsies, considered the gold standard for diagnosis, include multi-nucleated giant cells, necrotic tissue, and lymphocytic and fibroblast infiltration of the inflamed vessel wall. It is a disease seen primarily in the elderly and is reported as the most common systemic vasculitis in this age group. While the mortality rate in individuals with temporal arteritis is no different to that in individuals without the condition, its principle morbidity is the risk for permanent visual impairment. Upwards of 20–25% of patients with temporal arteritis suffer a permanent visual loss as a result. The prevalence of temporal arteritis in the general population has been estimated at somewhere between 22 and 24 per 100 000 women aged 50 years and older, while in men the prevalence is about one-third that value. The condition is considered rare under the age of 50.

While treatments are available that markedly decrease the likelihood of developing permanent visual loss, a clinical conundrum arises in that it can

Evidence-Based Emergency Care: Diagnostic Testing and Clinical Decision Rules. By J.M. Pines and W.W. Everett. Published 2008 by Blackwell Publishing, ISBN: 978-14051-5400-0.

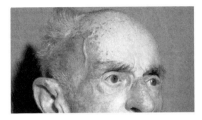

Figure 38.1 Giant cell arteritis. The superficial temporal artery is prominent and on palpation is found to be tender and pulseless, in an elderly male who has excruciating headaches and progressive impairment of vision. (Source: Wolff *et al. Fitzpatrick's Color Atlas and Synopsis of Clinical Dermatology* 4th Edition © 2001. Reproduced with permission of The McGraw-Hill Companies.)

be difficult to determine who should get a biopsy, which enables a diagnosis to be made. The time from the start of symptoms until biopsy-proven diagnosis ranges from one week to 1.5 years. Thus research has been sought to help determine historic features, signs and symptoms, and laboratory data that can be used to identify patients at high risk that should be referred for temporal artery biopsy.

Clinical question

"Which factors in a patient's history, physical examination, and laboratory values are predictive of having temporal arteritis?"

A pseudo meta-analysis performed in 2002 by Smetana and Shmerling examined history, physical examination, and laboratory test (ESR) findings that would accurately predict a diagnosis of temporal arteritis.[1] The authors maintained a strict requirement that only studies that enrolled patients that had undergone temporal artery biopsy to make the final diagnosis were included. Twenty-one studies involving 2680 patients were included and the prevalence of temporal arteritis was found to be 39%.

Two historic factors were identified that would raise a pre-test probability sufficiently to prompt additional investigation: jaw claudication (likelihood ratio (LR)+ 4.2; 95% CI: 2.8–6.2) and diplopia (LR+ 3.4; 95% CI: 1.3–8.6). Other symptoms commonly assessed that were positively associated with a diagnosis of temporal arteritis included headache of any type, anorexia, fever, weight loss, fatigue, myalgias, any visual symptoms, vertigo, and polymyalgia rheumatica. However, none had LRs that were sufficiency greater than 1.0 to be considered useful.

Two physical examination findings—beading of the temporal artery (LR+ 4.6; 95% CI: 1.1–18.4) and a prominent or enlarged temporal artery

(Fig. 38.1) (LR+ 4.3; 95% CI: 2.1–8.9)—were associated with a high likelihood of having biopsy-proven temporal arteritis. The absence of any temporal artery abnormality on physical examination had a sufficiently low negative LR to be clinically useful in lowering the suspicion of temporal arteritis (LR– 0.53; 95% CI: 0.38–0.75). Combinations of physical findings were not considered.

Finally, ESR data was clinically useful when the value was abnormal, with a negative LR value of 0.2 (95% CI: 0.08–0.51). ESR values in excess of 50 mm/h were also associated with a clinically useful negative LR value of 0.35 (95% CI: 0.18–0.67).

A prediction rule for identifying high-risk and low-risk patients using clinical features was generated in a study out of the Mayo Clinic.[2] The authors retrospectively collected history and physical examination findings, as well as ESR data, to build a predictive model for determining the need for a temporal artery biopsy. From 1988 to 1997 a total of 1113 patients suspected of having temporal arteritis underwent temporal artery biopsies. The diagnosis was confirmed in 33.5% of the cases. Table 38.1 shows the test characteristics for the most useful clinical elements (note that the 95% CIs were not provided in the original published report).

The authors used logistic regression modeling to derive a six-variable model to predict temporal arteritis, which included new headache, jaw claudication, scalp tenderness, ischemic optic neuropathy, age (in years), and ESR (in mm/h). Dichotomous variables received a scored of one if present

Table 38.1 Clinical and laboratory findings in the diagnosis of temporal arteritis from Younge et al.[2]

Clinical findings	Sensitivity, %	Specificity, %	PPV	NPV	LR+	LR–
New headache	67	60	46	79	1.7	1.8
Jaw claudication	40	94	78	76	6.7	1.6
Scalp tenderness	33	89	61	73	3	1.3
Jaw claudication + scalp tenderness	17	99	90	70	17	1.2
Headache + jaw claudication + scalp tenderness	15	99	90	70	15	1.2
Double vision	3.5	99	65	67	3.5	1.0
Abnormal ESR	99.6	16	33	99	1.2	40
Jaw claudication + double vision	2	100	100	67	n/a	0

ESR, erythrocyte sedimentation rate; LR, likelihood ratio; NPV, negative predictive value; PPV, positive predictive value.

and zero if absent. A formula was generated to enable the risk to be stratified into high, medium, and low categories as follows:

Score = −240 + 48*(headache) + 108*(jaw claudication) + 56*(scalp tenderness) + 1*(ESR) + 70*(ischemic optic neuropathy) + 1*(age)

A score of less than −110 was classified as being low risk, a score between −110 and 70 was classified as intermediate risk, and score above 70 was classified as being high risk. The authors report validating this scoring method on an independent set of 289 patients who also underwent temporal artery biopsy testing, but did not include any statistical details of its performance. To our knowledge, this scoring system has not been externally validated or replicated.

Comments

The diagnosis of temporal arteritis can be elusive and should be considered if a patient older than 50 years complains of any number of symptoms including headache, visual impairment or visual loss, scalp tenderness, or jaw claudication. Clinicians should maintain a cautious level of attentiveness given the long-term morbidity of permanent visual loss associated with temporal arteritis. Treatment considerations should be modified on the entirety of the clinicians' suspicion, based on the timing of the symptoms and any competing alternative diagnoses.

Unfortunately, as evidenced by the discussion above, there is no uniformity in predicting who is likely to have temporal arteritis and who does not. One line of commonality that is maintained is the value of an ESR test. While not highly specific, an abnormal ESR, as defined by the reference standard, is highly sensitive and is associated with useful negative LRs. Therefore, as this is an inexpensive, widely available laboratory test, it would be a reasonable one to obtain.

The studies used to generate these associations were retrospective in nature, and the reported associations represent findings from a highly selective group of patients—specifically those who actually underwent temporal artery biopsy. This form of verification bias, when only those patients in which there was a sufficiently high suspicion of the disease underwent the gold standard procedure, needs to be considered when applying and interpreting the findings in relation to unselected patients in an ED setting. While it is reasonable to extrapolate the results in concept, we do not recommend utilizing the scoring system or the reported likelihood score alone. Unfortunately, the low prevalence in the general population would require any prospective study examining predictive factors to enroll a prohibitive number of patients, many of whom would not ultimately undergo temporal artery biopsy.

Therefore, until a study using a large population database or registry can externally validate these reported findings, emergency physicians will need to rely on clinical judgment ultimately. However, a high suspicion of temporal arteritis in the presence of abnormal temporal artery findings, new headache, visual complaints, scalp tenderness, jaw claudication, or an abnormal ESR should prompt the clinician to consider consultation or referral for further evaluation.

References

1. Smetana, G.W. and Shmerling, R.H. (2002) Does this patient have temporal arteritis? *Journal of the American Medical Association* **287**(1): 92–101.
2. Younge, B.R., Cook, B.E., Bartley, G.B., Hodge, D.O. and Hunder, G.G. (2004) Initiation of glucocorticoid therapy: before or after temporal artery biopsy? *Mayo Clinic Proceedings* **79**: 483–491.

Chapter 39 **Intraocular Pressure**

Highlights

- Elevated intraocular pressure (IOP) is associated with glaucoma, the leading cause of blindness and visual impairment worldwide.
- The gold standard for measuring IOP in most studies is the Goldmann applanation tonometry; however, this is usually unavailable in the emergency department (ED)
- Schiotz and Tono-Pen tonometers are good screening tools in the ED enabling elevated IOP to be detected. However, they perform with variable accuracy compared to the gold standard and most commonly they underestimate IOP.

Background

Glaucoma is a leading cause of blindness and visual impairment worldwide. Patients may seek acute care for symptoms related to elevated intraocular pressure (IOP), which include not only eye pain, but visual impairment, nausea, vomiting, headaches, and abdominal pain. Measuring IOP is an essential component of evaluating patients suspected of having glaucoma, including both acute closed-angle and open-angle types, as well as blunt eye trauma and iritis (Fig. 39.1). Measurements above 20–22 mmHg are suspect and should prompt evaluation by an eye specialist either in the acute care setting or through urgent referral.

Different methods are available for measuring IOP and these are broadly divided into applanation and indentation tonometry methods, and non-contact (air puff) techniques. The Goldmann applanation tonometer is mounted on a slit lamp and consists of an applanation prism that comes into

---

Evidence-Based Emergency Care: Diagnostic Testing and Clinical Decision Rules. By J.M. Pines and W.W. Everett. Published 2008 by Blackwell Publishing, ISBN: 978-14051-5400-0.

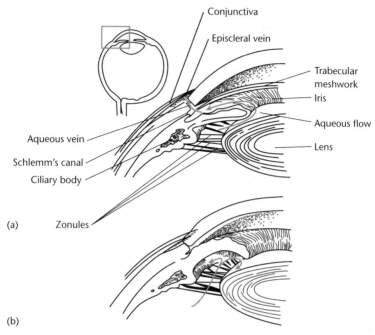

Figure 39.1 (a) Normal flow of aqueous from the ciliary body, through the pupil and out through the trabecular meshwork and Schlemm's canal, located in the anterior chamber angle. (b) Angle-closure glaucoma with pupillary block. Iris leaflet bows forward, blocking the chamber angle and prohibiting aqueous outflow. Meanwhile, aqueous production continues and intraocular pressure rises. (Source: Tintinalli *et al. Tintinalli's Emergency Medicine: A Comprehensive Study Guide* 6th Edition © 2004. Reproduced with permission of The McGraw-Hill Companies.)

contact with the patient's fluorescein-stained cornea using a cobalt-blue light filter, creating lighted semicircles. Correct alignment of the semicircles is translated into a pressure reading. The Goldmann applanation method has been accepted as the gold standard for most studies. The main limitation is that accurate readings are not possible with corneal irregularities, scarring, or edema. The most common indentation method uses the Tono-Pen XL tonometer. This is a handheld pen-like instrument that works by applying gentle indentations to the cornea to give electronic averaged readings of IOP (Fig. 39.2). The Tono-Pen is portable and utilizes a disposable rubber-condom tip cover making it ideal for the acute-care setting and for rapid sequential uses. The Schiotz tonometer is another common indentation method that uses a small weighted device to indent the cornea in the supine

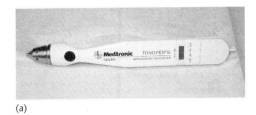

(a)

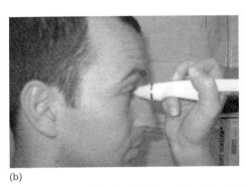

(b)

Figure 39.2 Tono-Pen tonometer (a) and positioning of the patient in the upright position for measurement of intraocular pressure using the Tono-Pen (b).

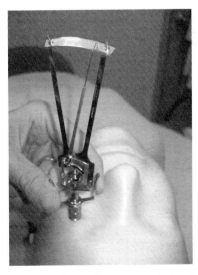

Figure 39.3 A Schiotz tonometer in use. The tonometer is placed gently onto the cornea while the patient is in the supine position.

patient (Fig. 39.3). The amount of indentation is measured against a calibrated weight and the IOP is then determined. Finally, there are non-contact methods that utilize puffs of air to flatten the cornea; the IOP is then calculated based on correlations of time to corneal flattening.

While the Goldmann applanation method has been accepted as the gold standard for most studies, most of us are not trained to use it. The equipment is bulky, non-portable, expensive, and is not widely available in acute care settings. Similarly, non-contact methods using puffs of air are cost prohibitive and not widely available in EDs. These limitations make the search for suitable alternatives to measure IOP in the acute care setting desirable. Schiotz tonometers and Tono-Pens are widely available and are usually within the budgetary constraints of most EDs.

Clinical question

"Are IOP measurements using the Schiotz tonometer or the Tono-Pen reliable and accurate compared to IOP measurements using the gold standard Goldmann applanation tonometry?"

Several small studies have compared IOP measurements using Goldmann tonometry to those using a Schiotz tonometer, the Tono-Pen, or both. Jackson and colleagues in Australia performed and analyzed serial IOP measurements in 72 patients using the Tono-Pen and the Schiotz tonometer.[1] Patients were recruited from a general practice, were over 50 years old, and had no prior history of glaucoma. IOP was first assessed by an ophthalmologist using a Goldmann tonometer, followed by measurements using the Schiotz tonometer and the Tono-Pen. An independent observer recorded the pressure reading and the physicians were blinded to the results. A total of 19 patients (26%) were found to have elevated IOP readings (≥21 mmHg), of which 18 received follow-up specialized eye care after the study. Only five of these had persistently elevated IOPs. The Schiotz tonometer was the most reliable instrument with 64–76% of IOP values falling to within 4 mmHg of those recorded using the gold standard method. Results using the Tono-Pen were extremely variable with 10–95% of values falling within 4 mmHg of those recorded using a Goldmann tonometer. Most measurements using the Tono-Pen tended to underestimate IOP. This study utilized three examining physicians and there was measurement variation by physicians with each method examined.

A small study out of Missouri examined IOP measurements with several portable tonometers, including the Tono-Pen and Schiotz tonometers, with Goldmann as the gold standard.[2] A total of 31 patients from a glaucoma clinic were enrolled and analyzed in the study (a total of 58 eyes were analyzed). The

Table 39.1 Results of intraocular pressure (IOP) measurement by tonometry (n = 58) from Wingert *et al.*[2]

Tonometer	Mean IOP (mmHg)	95% CI range (mmHg)	Standard error	Mean difference from Goldmann (mmHg)
Goldmann	18.2	—	0.8	—
Tono-Pen	15.8	7.7	0.6	2.5*
Schiotz	15.3	9.7	0.8	2.9*

* $P < 0.05$.

methods used for obtaining IOP measurements were standardized and the order of examinations was randomized following initial IOP measurements using Goldmann tonometry. Physicians were not blinded to the individual results from each method. Results shown in Table 39.1 illustrate that both Tono-Pen and Schiotz tonometers underestimated the IOP by 2–3 mmHg when compared to readings taken using the Goldmann tonometer.

In another small Australian study, researchers compared IOP measurements obtained using Tono-Pen and Goldmann tonometers to determine if measurements were similar (i.e. within 2 mmHg of each other).[3] A total of 138 patients were recruited from a glaucoma clinic; a further 22 patients were enrolled that had known elevated IOP. Among the 138 patients, IOPs ranged from 3 to 47 mmHg. Reproducibility of the results was excellent, as reflected in an intraclass correlation coefficient of 0.97 for the Goldmann tonometer and 0.95 for the Tono-Pen. Analysis of paired IOP readings revealed no statistical difference between methods (mean difference: right eyes = −0.4 mmHg, 95% CI: −6 − +5; left eyes = −0.3 mmHg, 95% CI: −5 − +5). When results were compared within three pressure ranges (0–10, 11–20, 20–≥30 mmHg), a divergence of agreement was shown for the high pressure readings. Results of IOP measurements for the 22 patients with known elevated pressures (range 24–58 mmHg) revealed a significant difference between methods (mean difference: −4.2 mmHg, 95% CI: −13 − +5), with the Tono-Pen consistently yielding lower values. These researchers concluded that while Tono-Pen measurements are reproducible, readings at higher IOPs may be underestimated.

British researchers compared IOP measurements using various methods in 105 patients from primary eye and glaucoma clinics.[4] Among the methods tested, Goldmann tonometry was the gold standard and the Tono-Pen method was the comparator (see Table 39.2). Methods were standardized across patients. The mean IOP reading obtained using the Tono-Pen tonometer was found to be 0.6 mmHg lower than Goldmann tonometry measurements, and this difference was consistent across a range of pressure values.

Table 39.2 Comparisons of intraocular pressure (IOP) measurements using Goldmann and Tono-Pen tonometry (n = 105) from Tonnu et al.[4]

Tonometer	Mean IOP (mmHg)	Range (mmHg)	Standard deviation	Mean difference from Goldmann (mmHg)
Goldmann	17.2	9–32	4.3	—
Tono-Pen	16.6	7–29	4.4	0.6*

* $P = 0.3$.

Comments

The clinical question of concern is whether portable, smaller, and more widely available instruments can be used to reliably and accurately measure IOP. These four studies confirm that the reliability of the Tono-Pen method is sound. That is, the results are reproducible across different users with acceptable minimal differences in the absolute pressure measurements obtained. While the data is not overwhelmingly convincing with regard to the reliability of the Schiotz tonometer, it is our opinion that it is unlikely to be worse than that of the Tono-Pen.

The issue of accuracy is more of a technical concern and appears to vary across studies. One study presented measured agreement to within 4 mmHg of the gold standard, while another study used a 2 mmHg difference as meaningful. It appears in some of the earlier studies that the Tono-Pen pressure readings were somewhat variable. More recent studies using the XL model indicate that measurements are reasonably accurate and do not differ significantly from those obtained using Goldmann tonometry. A trend within most studies, however, indicates that Tono-Pen measurements tend to underestimate IOP at high pressures, although this also appears to be minimized with the use of the XL model. Similar to the discussion of reliability, the accuracy of the Schiotz tonometer is not thought to differ greatly from that of the Tono-Pen. The Schiotz also tends to underestimate IOP measurements, but deciding on what constitutes a clinically significant difference from the gold standard is always a concern in studies. A 2 mmHg difference is seemingly negligible. However a 4 or 5 mmHg difference could significantly affect both the immediate and near future treatment.

Either the Tono-Pen or Schiotz tonometer should serve as a screening tool for patients suspected of having abnormal IOPs. However, both methods systematically underestimate IOP measurements when compared to the gold standard Goldmann tonometry method. Patients should be treated according to the timing, severity, and history of their symptoms as well as in relation to the measured IOP values. However, the diagnosis of ocular hypertension or glaucoma should not be excluded solely based on the IOP readings obtained in the ED. An emergent ophthalmology consult should be obtained when sufficient concern is raised by the treating physician and when elevated IOP measurements are reported. Borderline or normal IOP measurements should be referred for urgent eye evaluation by a specialist.

References

1. Jackson, C., Bullock, J., Pitt, M., Keogh, J., Glasson, W. and Hirst, L. (1995) Screening for glaucoma in a Brisbane general practice—the role of tonometry. *Australian and New Zealand Journal of Ophthalmology* **23**(3): 173–178.
2. Wingert, T.A., Bassi, C.J., McAlister, W.H. and Galanis, J.C. (1995) Clinical evaluation of five portable tonometers. *Journal of the American Optometric Association* **65**(11): 670–674.
3. Franzco, G.S.H., Byles, J., Franzco, J.L. and D'Este, C. (2004) Comparison of the Tono-Pen and Goldmann tonometer for measuring intraocular pressure in patients with glaucoma. *Clinical and Experimental Ophthalmology* **32**: 584–589.
4. Tonnu, P.A., Ho, T., Sharma, K., White, E., Bunce, C. and Garway-Heath, D. (2005) A comparison of four methods of tonometry: method agreement and inter-observer variability. *British Journal of Ophthalmology* **89**: 847–850.

Chapter 40 **Asthma**

Highlights

- Asthma is a common disease and is responsible for numerous emergency department (ED) visits and hospitalizations every year.
- Hospitalization rates are high for all asthmatics and relapse rates following ED visits are common among adults (~15%) and children (~10%).
- Global and specific clinical assessment factors are reliable among different providers caring for asthmatics in the ED.
- Numerous asthma scoring systems have been developed but few have been rigorously validated and replicated.
- The Pediatric Assessment Severity Score (PASS) is responsive and discriminates patients requiring admission from those that are stable for discharge, but its practical application has not been demonstrated.
- No uniform set of variables reliably predict the need for hospitalization or treatment relapse in adult asthmatics.

Background

Asthma is a chronic disease affecting over 16 million adults and 5 million children in the US alone, with nearly 20% requiring hospitalization annually. Worldwide it is estimated that there are over 300 million asthmatics.[1] Efforts to improve outpatient care for this disease have been promoted through the development of treatment guidelines, but many patients remain either undertreated or undiagnosed. Many patients with acute exacerbations of asthma receive their care in EDs. While the care for the asthmatic in the ED is fairly regimented, including bronchodilators and steroids, a certain percentage of asthmatics will require hospitalization and further inpatient care and

Evidence-Based Emergency Care: Diagnostic Testing and Clinical Decision Rules. By J.M. Pines and W.W. Everett. Published 2008 by Blackwell Publishing, ISBN: 978-14051-5400-0.

monitoring for their asthma flare. There have been multiple studies performed to try and predict which patients would require inpatient admission for acute asthma exacerbations or to predict the failure of outpatient therapy.

Clinical question

"Are there scoring systems for ED patients that predict asthma severity, the need for hospitalization, or relapses after treatment?"
Much of the medical literature on this topic is divided into pediatric and adult predictors and assessments for acute asthma. Therefore, the discussion will be presented in this way except for studies that included all age ranges, which will be discussed where appropriate.

Reproducibility of the clinical examination

In 2003 Stevens *et al.* examined the inter-rater reliability of the physical examination in children with asthma in order to address the concern that findings from clinical trials may not represent actual clinical practice because specially trained staff are usually involved.[2] Reproducibility of key physical findings and an overall global gestalt about the severity of the patient's condition by different people across different levels of training is the first step in establishing that a scoring system could be successfully developed and used clinically. The observers in this study included pediatric emergency physicians (n = 20), pediatric ED nurses (n = 50), and hospital respiratory therapists (n = 50). The observers received no prior specialized training on physical examination assessment for this study. Patients with acute asthma from a large urban children's hospital aged from 1 to 16 years were the examination subjects. Observers were asked to independently and simultaneously rate the following aspects on a scale of 1–3 or 1–4 on a standardized form: work of breathing, wheezing, decreased air entry, increased expiratory time, breathlessness, mental status, and respiratory rate. A global question assessing 'overall' severity with the options being asymptomatic, mild, moderate, or severe was also asked, and a composite score was calculated.

Weighted kappa statistics for each component of the examination for 230 pairs of examinations ranged from 0.61 to 0.74, while the overall severity (weighted kappa 0.80) and total scores (weighted kappa 0.82) had excellent agreement. Paired observers who were practitioners of the same profession had slightly better agreement for all elements assessed. The authors felt that this supported the use of structured and standardized formats to assess asthmatic pediatric patients. More reassuring was that among a diverse group of care providers a high level of agreement was found in the clinical assessment of acute asthmatics.

Severity scores in asthmatic children

Numerous pediatric asthma scores have been developed to assess the severity of the condition, including discriminative scores (aimed at gauging the severity at a single point in time), predictive scores (predicting particular outcomes), and evaluative scores (reflecting changes over time). Unfortunately, many were developed using small numbers of selected subjects, which had an impact on the generalizability of the results. For instance, of the 16 pediatric asthma scores as of 1994, 11 had sample sizes of less than 100, and only one included more than 300 study subjects.[3] More concerning and critical is that most were not and have not since been thoroughly evaluated with respect to accepted validation and performance measures. The handful that have undergone appropriate assessment usually included common sets of clinical findings with three to five items, with each item scored on a 0–2 or 0–3 scale.

In 2004 Gorelick *et al.* published a new pediatric asthma score—the PASS —that was developed and vigorously validated on a large, diverse pediatric asthma population with no exclusions based on severity or disposition (home or admission).[4] The score was validated and tested for reliability and responsiveness on a group of 1221 pediatric asthmatics in two EDs with an enrollment rate of 89% (out of 1379 eligible patients). Of these, 503 (41%) were admitted to an inpatient service. Clinical items examined during the study for inclusion in the final score had been included in prior clinical asthma scores and were deemed acceptable and pertinent (i.e. to have face validity) by the clinicians at the study sites. The final three-item score included an assessment of wheezing (none/mild, moderate, or severe/absent due to poor air exchange), work of breathing (none/mild, moderate, or severe), and prolongation of expiration (normal/mildly prolonged, moderately prolonged, or severely prolonged). Items assessed but not included in the final score were air entry, tachypnea, and mental status.

The three-item PASS score discriminated admitted versus discharged patients with a high level of confidence [area under the curve (AUC) values for the receiver operating characteristic (ROC) curves for each of the two EDs were 0.83 (95% CI: 0.8–0.86) and 0.85 (95% CI: 0.81–0.89)]. The new score was also responsive to changes (e.g. improvements) with serial assessments. Scores changed by 51–79% among those discharged home, whereas in those asthmatics admitted for inpatient care the scores changed by 25–32%. By comparison, the peak expiratory flow rate (PEFR) also changed by 25–32%, but the change was similar between admitted and discharged patients.

The PASS score has yet to be used in any new published studies. Its concept basis, rigorous testing, and validation may make it a useful tool, but it awaits more vigorous assessment before it can gain widespread acceptance for clinical use.

Predicting hospitalization in asthmatic children

A large prospective multicenter study by the Multicenter Airway Research Collaboration (MARC) Investigators examined risk factors and predictors for hospital admission among children aged 2 to 17 years that were seen in 44 EDs in 1997 and 1998.[5] Enrolling sites included 37 general hospitals and seven children's hospitals across 18 US states and four Canadian provinces. Data were prospectively collected 24 h per day for a median of two weeks. Repeat ED visits and patients discharged from the ED against medical advice were excluded.

A total of 1601 eligible children presenting to EDs with acute asthma were identified and 1178 patients were included in the analysis (74%). The admission rate was 23% (95% CI: 21–26) with an interquartile range of 11–31% across the 44 EDs. Multivariate logistic regression modeling produced patient variables that were independently predictive of hospital admission (Table 40.1). PEFR was not included in the logistic regression model because it was only able to be measured in 23% of the children. However, in the 23% of children that had PEFR measurements, those that were admitted had lower initial PEFRs compared to those that were not admitted (% predicted: 36 versus 50; mean difference: -13.7 (95% CI: $-13.8--13.6$). Demographic factors were not predictive of admission.

The MARC Investigators also examined the initial room air oxygen saturation reading to determine if, as a single variable, it could predict hospital admission in asthmatic children.[6] This study differed from prior studies in terms of both the number of enrolled patients and the multicenter study design, strengthening its generalizability. Initial oxygen saturation was documented for 1040 children with a mean reading of 95%. Admitted children had lower oxygen saturation levels compared to discharged patients (93 vs. 96%). The authors then used the initial oxygen saturation level to construct

Table 40.1 Independent predictors of hospital admission in children with asthma from multivariate logistic regression from Pollack et al.[5]

	Odds ratio	95% CI
Oxygen saturation (per decrease of 5%)	2.2	1.6–3.0
Number of inhaled beta-agonists during ED stay	2.1	1.8–2.4
Prior admission for asthma within past year	1.7	1.1–2.8
Pulmonary index score	1.3	1.1–1.4
Not taking corticosteroids at time of ED visit	0.3	0.2–0.6
No comorbidities	0.3	0.1–0.7

ED, emergency department.

multiple 2×2 tables of sensitivities and specificities for admission using different oxygen saturation level cut off points. An ROC curve plotting the sensitivity and 1–specificity values for predicting hospitalization in the study cohort was constructed, resulting in an AUC value of 0.76, which demonstrated only moderate discriminatory ability. The authors concluded that initial oxygen saturation is not a useful single predictor variable for hospital admission.

Treatment relapses in asthmatic children

Another large, prospective multicenter study by the MARC Investigators examined risk factors and predictors of treatment relapses among children age 2 to 17 years that were seen in 44 EDs in 1997 and 1998.[7] Enrolling sites included 37 general hospitals and seven children's hospitals. Only patients discharged from the ED were included. Data was prospectively collected 24 h per day over a median of two weeks. Telephone follow-ups were conducted two weeks after patient discharge to establish the rate of relapses, which was defined as any urgent visit to an ED as a result of another asthma attack.

A total of 1184 patients were enrolled with 303 excluded because they were hospitalized or had severe comorbid conditions. A total of 762 of the remaining 881 patients (86%) had complete follow-up and were included in the analysis. Relapse occurred in 10% (95% CI: 8–13) of children. There was no difference in the relapse rates between general and children's hospitals (12 vs. 10%). The four factors that were independently associated with relapse after multivariate analysis are shown in Table 40.2. The variables 'number of ED visits' and 'cigarette smoke exposure' were no longer significant when a separate analysis was performed looking only at relapses occurring within three days after ED discharge. There were no differences between relapse and no relapse patients during the initial ED visit with regard to symptom duration, treatment duration, treatment medications, or steroid prescription for home use.

Table 40.2 Independent predictors of treatment relapse in children with asthma from multivariate logistic regression from Emerman et al.[7]

	Odds ratio	95% CI
Asthma medication other than beta-agonists, steroids, cromolyn, or nedocromil	3.7	2.2–6.3
Age (for every 5 year increase)	1.4	1.0–1.8
Asthma related ED visits in past year (per 5 visits)	1.2	1.0–1.5
Cigarette smoke exposure	0.5	0.3–0.9

ED, emergency department.

Predicting hospitalization in asthmatics (children and adults)

Australian researchers asked whether a determination of asthma severity after 1 h of treatment in the ED is a better predictor of the need for admission compared to the initial assessment of asthma severity at ED presentation.[8] This observational cohort analyzed 720 patient presenting to 36 Australian EDs during a two-week period in 2001. Severity assessments at presentation and at 1 h, and dispositions were collected and compared. Clinical assessments of adult and pediatric patients followed the National Asthma Guidelines endorsed by the Australian National Asthma Campaign. The assessment had ratings of mild, moderate, and severe/life-threatening (with response meanings for each category) and included the following items: altered consciousness, physical exhaustion, talkativeness, pulsus paradoxus, central cyanosis, wheezing intensity, PEFR, forced expiratory volume in 1 sec (FEV_1; % predicted), pulse oximetry on presentation, and the need for admission.

Adults comprised 44% of the study cohort and overall 32% of patients required hospital admission. Among patients assessed as having mild asthma either at the initial presentation or after 1 h, more than 80% were able to be discharged home. Similarly, more than 85% of patients classified as severe at either of the assessments were admitted. A moderate rating at initial presentation was a poor predictor of the need for hospitalization. However, a moderate rating at the 1-h assessment predicted that 84% needed admission. The authors concluded that the response to therapy after 1 h for patients presenting to EDs with acute asthma is better than the initial severity assessment for predicting the need for hospital admission.

Predicting hospitalization in asthmatic adults

In another MARC study to examine patient characteristics associated with hospitalization for acute asthma, investigators used data collected from four prospective cohorts across 64 US and Canadian EDs with two-week telephone follow-ups.[9] The admission rate among the 1805 patients enrolled with complete data was 20% (95% CI: 18–22). Variables that were found to be independently associated with hospitalization are shown in Table 40.3. The multivariate model had an AUC value of 0.91, indicating excellent discrimination; however, no external validation of this model has been performed.

Researchers in 88 EDs across the US and Canada collected data during a median of two weeks from 1999 to 2002 as part of the MARC research alliance to study acute asthma. In an analysis of older versus younger adults presenting with acute asthma the investigators sought to examine differences in asthma severity, treatments, and outcomes.[10] Ages were divided into three groups: 18–34, 35–54, and 55 years or above. Patients reporting a history of

Table 40.3 Independent predictors of hospitalization in adults with asthma from multivariate logistic regression from Weber et al.[9]

	Odds ratio	95% CI
Use of home nebulizers*	2.7	1.6–4.5
Final peak flow (per decrease of 10% predicted)	2.6	2.2–3.1
Female sex	2.1	1.3–3.6
Asthma medication other than beta-agonists or inhaled corticosteroids*	1.9	1.2–3.0
Beta-agonist treatment in the ED	1.4	1.3–1.6
Initial peak flow (per increase of 10% predicted)	1.4	1.2–1.7
Initial respiratory rate (per 5 breaths)	1.3	1.1–1.7

ED, emergency department.
*During the past four weeks.

chronic obstructive pulmonary disease (chronic bronchitis or emphysema) or who had a smoking history in excess of 10 pack-years were excluded. Patient follow-ups were made by telephone interview two weeks after the ED visit.

The study enrolled 2064 patients (84% of those eligible), of whom 56% were in the youngest age category and 6% were in the oldest age category. Overall 348 patients (17%) required hospital admission. Significantly higher admission rates occurred with increasing age categories (13% in youngest, 19% in middle, 38% in oldest age groups). The seriousness of the acute asthma condition at the time of ED presentation, based on initial PEFR (% predicted), was severe for all groups (median 47%). Multivariate modeling revealed that patients aged 55 year or above had the poorest response to bronchodilator treatments after controlling for demographic and severity factors. In a logistic regression model that excluded the change in the PEFR, increasing age was an independent predictor of hospital admission. This association was eliminated when the change in the PEFR was included in the model (Table 40.4).

Data for the two-week follow-up was presented for 64% of all patients. This demonstrated that patients aged 55 years or above were hospitalized longer (median stay two, three, and four days for the 18–34, 35–54, and ≥55 age groups, respectively) and were more likely to have relapses in the two weeks following the initial ED visit (12, 19, and 25% for the 18–34, 35–54, and ≥55 age groups, respectively).

Treatment relapses in asthmatic adults

Using the MARC Investigators data collected between 1996 and 1997, Emerman et al. examined the factors associated with relapses among adult

Table 40.4 Independent predictors of hospitalization in adult asthmatics from multivariate logistic regression from Banerji et al.[10]

	Odds ratio (95% CI) of need for hospitalization		
	Age 18–35*	Age 35–54	Age ≥55
Model[#] excluding PEF change	1.0	1.2 (0.8–1.7)	2.0 (1.2–3.4)
Model[#] including PEF change	1.0	1.2 (0.8–2.0)	0.9 (0.4–2.1)

PEF, peak expiratory flow.
* Reference category.
[#] Model included variables shown in Table 40.3.

asthmatics following treatment for acute asthma.[11] Among the 641 patients enrolled, a total of 17% reported a relapse during the two weeks following the initial ED visit. The initial, final, and change in PEFR values were no different between patients who did and did not relapse. Multivariate logistic regression modeling found that duration of symptoms lasting 1–7 days [odds ratio (OR) 2.5; 95% CI: 1.2–5.2], use of home nebulizers (OR 2.2; 95% CI: 1.5–3.9), multiple urgent care visits for asthma (OR 1.4; 95% CI: 1.5–3.9), and multiple ED visits for asthma (OR 1.3; 95% CI: 1.5–1.5) were all independent predictors associated with relapse after controlling for age, sex, race, primary care provider status, and number of reported asthma triggers.

Comments

Asthma is a prevalent disease that is responsible for many ED visits and hospitalizations. Numerous asthma scoring systems have been developed, primarily in the pediatric literature. However, few have been vigorously derived and validated, and none have gained widespread acceptance. While the clinical assessment of acute asthmatics has been shown to be reproducible, we cannot at this time recommend any particular scoring system. The PASS appears to meet the basic criteria for a successful scoring tool in that it: (i) has sound derivation and validation using a broad group of unselected study subjects; (ii) uses a limited number of clinically relevant items; and (iii) has been shown to be discriminative and responsive. However, its use has not been reported outside of the derivation/validation studies and, while the PASS is a tool intended for use in pediatric patients, no similar tool exists for adult asthma. Is a separate tool necessary? This would be an ideal topic for further study.

Studies have examined sets of predictors of particular outcomes including discharge, hospitalization, and treatment relapse. In children, no set of demographic variables reliably predicts hospital admission. Historic and clinical factors found to be predictive of hospitalization include low initial oxygen saturation, the extent of beta-agonist use in the ED (i.e. total number of nebulizer treatments given), prior admissions for asthma in the previous year, and the absence of comorbidities or steroid use at the time of the ED visit. Assessment of the need for hospitalization after 1 h of treatment in the ED appears to be a better predictor of hospitalization compared with the initial assessment because some patients will improve rapidly following treatment. For patients that are treated and discharged, the relapse rate remains high (≥10% in children) and this is associated with the use of asthma medications other than routine medications, as well as with the annual number of asthma-related ED visits. Among adult asthmatics, several variables appear to predict hospitalization but none are consistent across studies. Similarly, relapse after treatment in adult asthmatics (>16%) is associated with duration of symptoms, self treatment at home, and the extent of prior urgent care and ED visits related to asthma.

Overall, no uniform set of predictor variables is able to reliably predict the outcomes of need for hospitalization or treatment relapse. Some variables such as prior admissions, extent of pharmacologic treatment prior to the ED visit, and evaluation after a period of treatment in the ED are intuitive elements that should impact your decision to admit or discharge a patient. The largest diverse collection of studies examining acute asthmatics, from the MARC Investigators, as well as the promising development of the PASS, add breadth and depth to the discussion, yet further studies are certainly warranted. Perhaps sets of factors within subgroups of adult asthmatics can be identified that will be predictive as well as responsive indictors for clinical use, much in the same way that pediatric scores have been developed separately from adult predictors. Finally, improvements in therapy will necessitate refinements in any prediction tool. We should continue to base patient disposition on the clinical assessment after a short period of intense treatment in the ED. But additional elements warrant consideration including issues surrounding access to care, access to appropriate medications, and environmental factors, few of which have been incorporated into the clinical studies performed to date.

References

1. Masoli, M., Fabian, D., Holt, S. and Beasley, R., and for the Global Initiative for Asthma (GINA) Program. (2004) The global burden of asthma: executive summary of the GINA Dissemination Committee report. *Allergy* **59**: 469–478.
2. Stevens, M.W., Gorelick, M.H. and Schultz, T. (2003) Interrater agreement in the clinical evaluation of acute pediatric asthma. *Journal of Asthma* **40**(3): 311–315.

3. van der Windt, D.A. (1994) Clinical scores for acute asthma in pre-school children – a review of the literature. *Journal of Clinical Epidemiology* **47**(6): 635–646.
4. Gorelick, M.H., Stevers, M.W., Schultz, T.R. and Scribano, P.V. (2004) Performance of a novel clinical score, the Pediatric Asthma Severity Score (PASS), in the evaluation of acute asthma. *Academic Emergency Medicine* 11(1): 10–18.
5. Pollack, C.V., Pollack, E.S., Baren, J.M., *et al.*, and for the Multicenter Airway Research Collaboration Investigators. (2002) A prospective multicenter study of patient factors associated with hospital admission from the emergency department among children with acute asthma. *Archives of Pediatrics and Adolescent Medicine* **156**: 934–940.
6. Keahey, L., Bulloch, L., Becker, A.B., Pollack, C.V., Clark, S. and Camargo, C.A., and for the Multicenter Airway Research Collaboration (MARC) Investigators. (2002) Initial oxygen saturation as a predictor of admission in children presenting to the emergency department with acute asthma. *Annals of Emergency Medicine* **40**(3): 300–307.
7. Emerman, C.L., Cydulka, R.K., Crain, E.F., Rowe, B.H., Radeos, M.S. and Camargo, C.A., and for the MARC Investigators. (2001) Prospective multicenter study of relapse after treatment for acute asthma among children presenting to the emergency department. *Journal of Pediatrics* **138**(3): 318–324.
8. Kelly, A.M., Kerr, D. and Powell, C. (2004) Is severity assessment after one hour of treatment better for predicting the need for admission in acute asthma? *Respiratory Medicine* **98**: 777–781.
9. Weber, E.J., Silverman, R.A., Callaham, M.L., *et al.* (2002) A prospective multicenter study of factors associated with hospital admission among adults with acute asthma. *American Journal of Medicine* **113**: 371–378.
10. Banerji, A., Clark, S., Afilalo, M., Blanda, M.P., Cydulka, R.K. and Camargo, C.A. (2006) Prospective multicenter study of acute asthma in younger versus older adults presenting to the emergency department. *Journal of the American Geriatrics Society* **54**(1): 48–55.
11. Emerman, C.L., Woodruff, P.G., Cydulka, R.K., Gibbs, M.A., Pollack, C.V. and Camargo, C.A., and for the MARC Investigators. (1999) Prospective multicenter study of relapse following treatment for acute asthma among adults presenting to the emergency department. *Chest* **115**(4): 919–927.

Index

Page numbers in *italics* refer to figures; those in **bold** to tables.